Me[illegible] Postmenopause and Ageing

Guest Editor: Louis Keith

[illegible]ditors: Margaret Rees and [illegible]r

BRITISH MENOPAUSE SOCIETY
Meeting the Challenge of Menopause

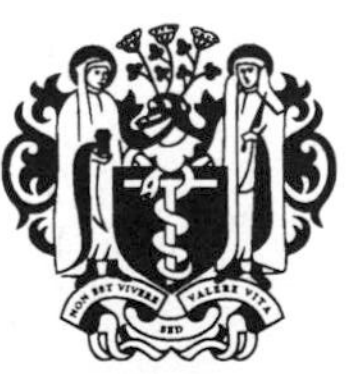

The ROYAL SOCIETY of MEDICINE PRESS Limited

Published by the Royal Society of Medicine Press Ltd
1 Wimpole Street, London W1G 0AE, UK
Tel: +44 (0) 20 7290 2921
Fax: +44 (0) 20 7290 2929
Email: publishing@rsm.ac.uk
Website: www.rsmpress.co.uk

British Library Cataloguing in Publication Data

A catalogue record for this book is available from the British Library
ISBN 1 85315 660 4

Distribution in Europe and Rest of World:
Marston Book Services Ltd
PO Box 269
Abingdon
Oxon OX14 4YN, UK
Tel: +44 (0) 1235 465500
Fax: +44 (0) 1235 465555
Email: direct.order@marston.co.uk

Distribution in the USA and Canada:
Royal Society of Medicine Press Ltd
c/o Jamco Distribution Inc.
1401 Lakeway Drive
Lewisville TX 75057, USA
Tel: +1 800 538 1287
Fax: +1 972 353 1303
Email: jamco@majors.com

Distribution in Australia and New Zealand:
Elsevier Australia
30–52 Smidmore Street
Marrickville NSW 2204
Australia
Tel: + 61 2 9517 8999
Fax: + 61 2 9517 2249
Email: service@elsevier.com.au

British Menopause Society (registered charity no. 10151440),
4–6 Eton Place, Marlow, Bucks, SL7 2QA, UK www.the-bms.org

Designed and Typeset by Phoenix Photosetting, Chatham, Kent
Printed and bound by Krips b.v., Meppel, The Netherlands

List of contents

About the editors

Louis Keith is Emeritus Professor of Obstetrics and Gynecology at the Feinberg School of Medicine, Northwestern University, Chicago. He is a Fellow of the American College of Obstetricians and Gynecologists, Editor-in-Chief of the International Journal of Fertility and Women's Medicine and Assistant Editor of the International Journal of Gynecology and Obstetrics.

Margaret Rees is a Medical Gynaecologist and Reader in Reproductive Medicine in the Nuffield Department of Obstetrics and Gynaecology, University of Oxford. She runs the menopause clinic in Oxford – one of the first established in the UK. She is the editor in chief of the *Journal of the British Menopause Society* and an expert advisor to Women's Health Concern.

Tony Mander is a practising Consultant Gynaecologist, is deputy editor of the *Journal of the British Menopause Society* and honorary clinical teacher in Obstetrics and Gynaecology at Manchester University. He is currently President of the forum of food and health at the Royal Society of Medicine and is an expert advisor to Women's Health Concern.

List of contributors

Catrina Bain
Specialist Registrar in Obstetrics and Gynaecology, Division of Developmental Medicine, University of Glasgow, Glasgow, UK

Bob Barber
Honorary Clinical Senior Lecturer and Consultant Old Age Psychiatrist, Institute of Ageing and Health, Newcastle General Hospital, Newcastle, UK

Sylvia M Botros
Northwestern University Medical School, Chicago, Illinois, USA

Sarah Daley
Specialist Registrar, Institute of Ageing and Health, Newcastle General Hospital, Newcastle, UK

Tom Dening
Medical Director, Cambridgeshire & Peterborough Mental Health Partnership NHS Trust, Huntingdon, Cambridgeshire, UK

William D Fraser
Head of Metabolic Bone Disease Unit, Department of Clinical Chemistry and Metabolic Medicine, Royal Liverpool University Hospital, Liverpool, UK

Roger P Goldberg
Assisstant Professor, Northwestern University Medical School, Chicago, Illinois, USA; Director of Urogynecology Research, Evanston Continence Center, Evanston, Illinois, USA

Rebecca Hardy
Senior Research Scientist, Medical Research Council, National Survey of Health and Development; Honorary Senior Lecturer, Department of Epidemiology and Public Health, Royal Free and University College Medical School, London, UK

Jean Hodson
General Practitioner, Bridge House Medical Centre, Stratford upon Avon, Warwickshire, UK

Sakeba N Issa
Clinical Research Fellow, Feinberg School of Medicine, Northwestern University, Chicago, Illinois, USA

Louis Keith
Emeritus Professor of Obstetrics and Gynecology, Feinberg School of Medicine, Northwestern University, Chicago, Illinois, USA; The Center for the Study of Multiple Births, Chicago, Illinois, USA

Diana Kuh
Senior Research Scientist, Medical Research Council, National Survey of Health and Development; Professor of Life Course Epidemiology, Department of Epidemiology and Public Health, Royal Free and University College Medical School, London, UK

Guy WL Lloyd
Consultant Cardiologist, East Sussex NHS Trust, Eastbourne General Hospital, East Sussex, UK

Alisoun Milne
Senior Lecturer in Social Gerontology, Tizard Centre, School for Social Policy, Sociology & Social Research, University of Kent, UK

Gita Mishra
Women's Health Research Fellow, Medical Research Council, National Survey of Health and Development; Senior Research Fellow, Department of Epidemiology and Public Health, Royal Free and University College Medical School, London, UK

John O'Brien
Professor of Old Age Psychiatry, Institute of Ageing and Health, Newcastle General Hospital, Newcastle, UK

Peter K Sand
Northwestern University Medical School, Chicago, Illinois, USA

Leena Sharma
Associate Professor of Medicine, Feinberg School of Medicine, Northwestern University, Chicago, Illinois, USA

Wasing Taggu
Registrar in Cardiology, East Sussex NHS Trust, Eastbourne District General Hospital, East Sussex, UK

Matthew Walters
Honorary Consultant Physician, Division of Cardiovascular and Medical Sciences, Western Infirmary, Glasgow, UK

Lawrence Whalley
Crombie Ross Professor of Mental Health, Institute of Applied Health Sciences, School of Medicine, University of Aberdeen, Aberdeen, UK

Preface

From childhood onwards, we repeatedly hear the truly ancient aphorism, 'Time marches onward' without giving it much thought. Today, however, sufficient data exist to require that this phrase be modified to reflect our increasing knowledge of the events taking place around us. In reality, the wording should now be ' Time marches on and the population is ageing'. Indeed, by 2050 it is projected that there will be three times as many elderly people as today and the over 65s will comprise an astonishing 17% of the world's population. The global implications of this are enormous, staggering and potentially catastrophic. Specifically, from the point of view of the readership of this book, as women tend to live longer than men their medical needs will become a significant public health issue. It is not surprising, therefore, that postmenopausal health problems, arising not only from ageing, but also from oestrogen deficiency, are 'hot topics' for medical professionals from a wide variety of healthcare disciplines and allied services.

Menopause, postmenopause and ageing discusses how specific postmenopausal health problems are thought to arise, and what are today's most promising treatment options. In addition, it describes the provision of home and residential care for older women in relation to their medical conditions. Health problems in the elderly comprise genetic as well as environmental components, with 'wanna-be' centenarians having a different health profile from those who die young. Common problems include dementia, stroke, myocardial infarction, osteoporosis, osteoarthritis and urinary incontinence. When disease accumulation is sufficient, home care becomes an increasingly important aspect of the global plan to access contact with appropriate caregivers. This may require coordination of the efforts of members of a multidisciplinary care team in order to maintain some degree of independence. With increasing frailty residential care is often required. In either instance, the conditions that lead to the need for out-of-home placement do not disappear, but often worsen as the new resident adjusts to their new foreign surroundings.

The aim of this book is to provide a concise guide (suitable for a multidisciplinary team) on the management of health problems after the menopause. International experts have written the chapters. At the end of each chapter a further reading list of relevant publications completes and augments the preceding discussion.

Louis Keith
Margaret Rees
Tony Mander

1 Genetic determinants of disease in later life

Lawrence Whalley

Introduction

A general decline in physiological functioning is the hallmark of ageing. As regulatory systems age, they are more easily perturbed by stressors, show a greater amplitude of stress responses and after stress take longer to return to baseline or resting levels. Together with reduced efficiency of immunological surveillance, these changes characterize the ageing processes. By themselves, the age-related regulatory changes in many biological systems appear to explain the increase of many complex diseases with age.

Behind this simple idea is the suggestion that these apparently diverse ageing processes share common genetic and environmental determinants. From an historical perspective, theories of ageing have now moved away from the central idea, usually attributed to Charles Darwin, that ageing is a non-adaptive process – an unavoidable property of all living tissue – to the proposal that ageing is a genetically determined disease with its own 'ageing' genes that regulate critical biochemical pathways. These new concepts support the idea that the identification of ageing processes common to many, if not all, age-related diseases may lead to interventions that postpone ageing and thus delay the onset of age-related diseases.

Age-related or age-dependent?

Dementia, cardiovascular disease, cerebrovascular disease, chronic obstructive pulmonary disease (COPD), osteoporosis and certain cancers comprise the majority of common age-related diseases (Figure 1.1 and Table 1.1). These conditions are major causes of death and disability worldwide and, as life

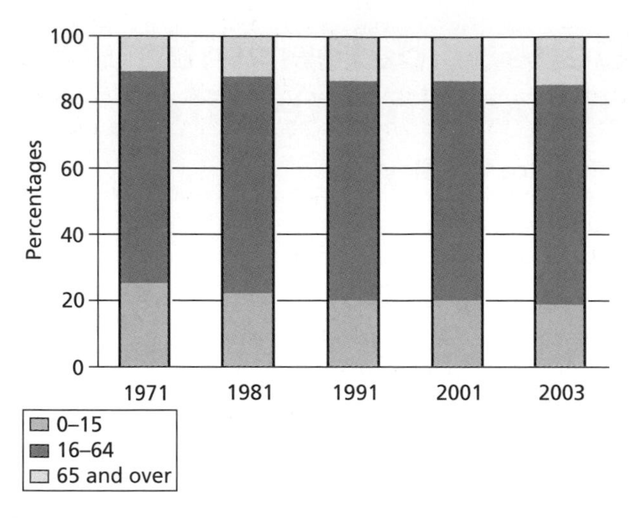

Figure 1.1 Population by age – 16% of UK population are aged 65 or over

Table 1.1

Causes of mortality in women, 2002 in England and Wales.

	Age				
Condition	**50–59**	**60–69**	**70–79**	**80–89**	**>90**
Ischaemic heart disease ICD-10 I20-I25	1097	3682	11,903	19,990	9010
Cerebrovascular disease ICD-10 I60-69	707	1610	6955	16,938	9795
Dementia ICD-10 FO1,FO3	10	94	1046	4413	3573
Chronic obstructive pulmonary disease ICD-10 J40-44	391	1325	4197	3958	1053
Colon cancer ICD-10 C18	308	688	1492	1662	485
Cancer (bronchus and lung) ICD-10 C34	1242	2308	4395	2698	376
Breast cancer ICD-10 C50	1871	2027	2658	2605	1055
Osteoporosis with pathological fracture ICD-10 M 80	3	13	105	478	426

See www.statistics.gov.uk

expectancy increases in the developed world, they make increasing personal and economic demands on contemporary societies. While all of these conditions are age-related, it is unclear if they are age-dependent. This is of potential causal importance and is certainly relevant to the discussion of possible genetic causes.

If increased incidence with age depends on underlying intrinsic ageing processes, and ageing itself has precise genetic determinants, then it may be reasonable to assume that some of that genetic contribution is shared between some, if not most, age-related diseases. In technical language this would be subsumed under the phrase '*common cause hypothesis of genetic contributions to age-related diseases and to ageing processes*' and was eloquently articulated in a study of cognitive ageing by Christensen and her colleagues in 2001. If biological parameters that are known to change consistently with ageing (examples are forced expiratory volume, grip strength, balance, visual acuity) could be combined to provide a measure of biological age, it might be shown that individuals differed in their rates of biological ageing. These variations might then explain individual differences in susceptibility to age-related diseases and instead these conditions could be considered as age-dependent. So far, differences in rates of biological ageing do not reliably distinguish between persons matched for calendar age, with and without specific age-related non-cognitive conditions.

Heritability of ageing and age-related diseases

Studies of age-related diseases suggest that their heritability is similar to current estimates of the heritability of life expectancy. Population-based and twin studies of late-onset disorders, such as Alzheimer's disease, cancer, osteoporosis, cardiovascular disease and chronic obstructive pulmonary disease, indicate that a significant genetic component is present in each of them – heritability is calculated to be in the range of 30–40%. Most reviews of life expectancy rely on Scandinavian twin studies that estimate its heritability at about 20–30%. The overall impression is that non-inherited, largely environmental factors are major determinants of life expectancy and common age-related diseases. Nevertheless, this does not imply that genes are unimportant. Modern molecular genetic techniques have identified mutations in familial forms of Alzheimer's disease (AD), Parkinson's disease (PD) and autosomal dominant macular atrophy (adMO), which help unravel the molecular mechanisms of disease in more common, sporadic late-onset forms of these diseases. Data derived by these techniques should not mask the fact that heritability estimates, especially of life expectancy, indicate that genetic contributions to ageing and age-related diseases are probably complex and that the contributions of individual genes are weak.

Ageing genes

If genes that convey longevity could be discovered, then these may be relevant to age-related diseases. This possibility rests on the likelihood that:

- these genes reduce susceptibility to age-related diseases, especially in extreme old age
- these genes may modify cellular and biochemical pathways involved in mechanisms of age-related disease (see Table 1.2).

The best-known example of this is the ε4 allele of the apolipoprotein E gene that decreases in frequency with advancing age, whereas the much rarer ε2 allele becomes more frequent. These findings are attributed to increased mortality in AD and cardiovascular diseases associated with the ε4 allele and the slight protection afforded by the ε2 allele. The siblings and children of centenarians show reduced rates of age-related cardiovascular diseases, hypertension, diabetes and stroke but not osteoporosis, cancers and thyroid disease, suggesting that genetic effects, in addition to apoE polymorphisms, are greater in the former disease group than the latter in whom environmental effects may predominate.

Whilst the exact identity of 'longevity genes' is unknown, much current thinking concerns genes regulating inflammatory processes. This notion is supported by repeated observations that age-related diseases (like AD, PD, atherosclerosis and type 2 diabetes) are sometimes initiated or exacerbated by

Table 1.2
Longevity and ageing genes

1. Genes that cause ageing (P53?).
2a. Genes that increase the risk of a specific illness early in life but do not apper to be related to ageing (eg cystic fibrosis and CF gene).
2b. Genes that alter longevity because they increase the risk of a specific illness early in life whose features resemble, to some extent, some of the consequences of aging (eg Werners gene).
3. Genes that influence or cause age-related illnesses (eg Alzheimer's disease and Apolipoprotein E ε-4).
4. Low-fitness genes that extend maximum life-span, probably by slowing down aging (as observed in lower organism mutations, eg daf genes).
5. Polymorphic genetic loci that influence the rate of ageing (many quantitative trait loci with varying influence: on ageing and age-associated diseases).
6. Genes that influence differences in life-span among species (eg longevity enabling genes).

Adapted from: Miller RA, Science of Aging Knowledge Environment 2001 systemic inflammation. This has supported the proposition that an 'anti-inflammatory genotype' is linked to longevity. Candidate genes have included the anti-inflammatory interleukin-10 (*IL-10*) and the pro-inflammatory tumour necrosis factor-α–308 (*TNFα-308*) in which polymorphisms are functionally important, increasing and decreasing levels of TNF-α. Inflammatory processes are also implicated in arthritis, AD, cancer and atherosclerosis. A link between cancer and inflammation was suspected because epidemiological studies had shown that the risk of cancer is increased when tissues are chronically inflamed and long-term use of non-steroidal anti-inflammatory drugs (NSAIDs) reduces the risk of several cancers. Furthermore, histology of tumour masses reveal numerous cell types, including many non-malignant cells such as those involved in the inflammatory response. Communication between malignant cells and inflammatory cells takes place through unknown pathways that probably include pro-inflammatory cytokines, such as TNF-α (above) and the gene transcription factor NF-κB. These interactions may prove relevant to understanding genetic determinants of increased age-related susceptibility to several types of cancer.

Linkage analysis

No consensus exists on the optimal approach to the identification of ageing genes or genetic determinants of late-onset diseases. Linkage analysis aims to map the genetic locus of a gene contributing to susceptibility to a disease through precisional cloning. The analysis begins with a map of polymorphic DNA markers whose chromosomal position is known. Within affected families (pedigrees) these polymorphisms are examined to determine which, if any, co-segregate with the disease. Pedigrees are then carefully examined to see if co-segregation could have arisen by chance; this is usually expressed as a lod score. The next stage requires detailed examination of genes in and around the chromosomal locus of the linked polymorphism (positional cloning). This process is greatly assisted when a chromosomal map of the area is available and the functions of neighbouring genes are known. When the function of a nearby gene can be plausibly linked to the pathogenesis of the disease, then this becomes a candidate gene and so stimulates intense research efforts.

This method is used extensively in genetic studies of age-related disorders. There are, however, limitations with this approach. Few, if any, common age-related diseases are attributable to the effects of a single gene. Also, because the parents and siblings of index cases of age-related disease are also aged, potentially informative samples are reduced by death. Nevertheless, linkage analyses have paid huge dividends in AD research. The neuropathology of AD is characterized by deposition of amyloid fibrils and aggregates, neurofibrillary tangles and neuronal death. Early onset forms of AD are caused by mutations in the amyloid precursor protein gene (*APP*) or in the presenilin genes (*PS1* and *PS2*). Identification of the biochemical pathways involved has given insights into the pathogenesis of early onset AD that are probably relevant to late onset forms but, so far, these specific mutations have not been shown to account for more than 0.03% of cases of late onset AD.

Genes, healthy behaviour and ageing

The ability to remain independent, find food and warmth, and to maintain social relationships is jeopardized by ageing. A healthy central nervous system is essential to the acquisition and maintenance of these survival-promoting behaviours and is a necessary component of successful ageing. It is reasonable, therefore, to conjecture that genes determining susceptibility to age-related diseases may share properties with genes that enhance acquisition of adaptive behaviours (especially in later life) and with genes that help us adapt to stressors (like illnesses or lack of food).

At first, it seems an impossible task to detect what these genes might be. But studies in lower animals have identified genes that control lifespan and also regulate resistance to stress. One such biochemical pathway is stimulated by insulin-like proteins and another by serotonin. The most remarkable finding from studies on the genetics of ageing has been the substantial similarities in genes that control life span in yeast, worms, fruitflies and mammals. In the roundworm *Caenorhabditis elegans* and the fruitfly *Drosophila melanogaster,* insulin-like signalling controls lifespan and recently studies in mice provided similar results. Benefits of ageing genes extend to increased resistance to oxidative damage and heat shock. Perhaps this indicates that increased longevity is tightly linked to the ability to repair diverse types of cellular damage.

Brain-derived neurotrophic factor (BDNF) is interesting because of its relevance to learning, energy metabolism and the stress response. It has many insulin-like properties in the brain together with important roles in the integration of sensory information in stress responses and in support of homeostatic mechanisms. Serotonin has similar roles in control of appetitive behaviours and in the sleep–wake cycle, which is implicated in susceptibility to age-related diseases (especially obesity and depressive disorders). These signalling molecules and insulin-like signalling through insulin and insulin growth factor 1 (IGF-1) are important in the regulation of glucose metabolism, and impaired regulation (through insulin resistance) is central to the 'metabolic syndrome' which contributes to the risks of late onset cardiovascular disease and diabetes. Actions of insulin/IGF1 and its receptor in the brain are important in synaptic plasticity (the basis of learning) and can mitigate the effects of brain oxidative stress, ischaemia and AD.

BDNF has many properties shared with insulin and insulin-like proteins. It can help protect neurons against injury and is intimately involved in neurodevelopment. With ageing, as with insulin-like proteins, there is decreased brain BDNF and decreased efficiency of responses to stress. It is possible that the regulation of stress responses was highly conserved in evolution and that such regulation involves mechanisms that control glucose metabolism, stress resistance, susceptibility to age-related diseases and life span.

Gene–environment interactions

Measures of dietary exposure are the most commonly investigated environmental factors in the study of gene–environment interactions in ageing and age-related diseases. There are four main ways in which genes and nutrients may interact:

- nutrients may up- or down-regulate gene transcription
- nutrients or dietary components may damage DNA
- nutrients may protect DNA from damage
- nutrients may be involved in genetic 'programming' of metabolic pathways.

Studies of these topics are in their infancy but important findings are already available.

Specific polymorphisms in genes relating to vitamin B_{12} metabolism [eg methylene tetrahydrofolate reductase (c677T and a1298C), methionine synthase (A2756G), methionine synthase reductase (A66G), transcobalamin (G776C) and cystathionine α-synthase (68 base pair insertion at base 844)] can be related to vascular health in certain individuals and may interact with polymorphisms elsewhere (eg APOε4). Hyperhomocysteinuria is linked to increased risk of several age-related disorders, including stroke, osteoporosis and Alzheimer's disease. These specific polymorphisms may account for some of the differences between individuals in plasma homocysteine concentrations. The general principle seems to be that the single-gene–phenotype model is rarely fruitful and that it is important to study multiple combinations of genes.

DNA damage is linked to several late onset diseases including some cancers and Alzheimer's disease. Antioxidant defences help combat DNA damage either through the actions of specific enzymes (eg superoxide dismutases) or through extrinsic dietary antioxidants, such as α-tocopherol or the carotenoids. Increased dietary intake of these nutrients can reduce the increased leucocyte DNA damage (detected by the Comet assay) associated with tobacco smoking.

Nutritional programming during critical periods of development may affect susceptibility to late onset diseases (Figure 1.2). At first this hypothesis was considered from the point of view of caloric malnutrition and sub-optimal fetal growth. However, the proposition is now finding support among those who study the effects of specific nutrients on varied developmental pathways. The underlying proposition remains relatively unchanged – essentially, the maternal nutritional environment during pregnancy provides the developing fetus with key information about the likely nutritional environment that will be encountered in maturity. Obviously, such 'nutritional priming' must be confined to a critical time in development otherwise later brief exposures to malnutrition may have unwanted effects on reproduction and survival. Individuals exposed to a poorly nourished fetal environment anticipate further privations and adapt genetically to food shortages by conserving glucose through the acquisition of insulin resistance. This adaptive strategy is successful but can prove disastrous if the adult environment is nutrient- and energy-rich. The mismatched offspring then develops the features of the metabolic syndrome (abdominal obesity, hypercholesterolaemia, hyperglycaemia and hypertension) and is prone to late onset diabetes and ischaemic heart disease.

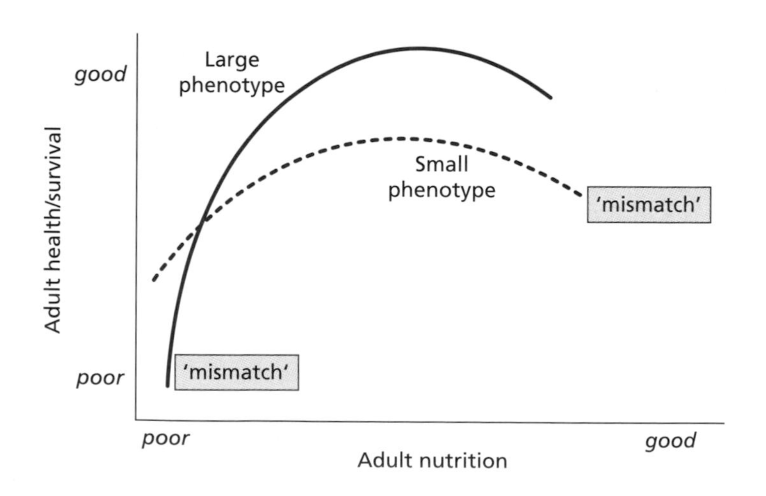

Figure 1.2 Adult health programmed by fetal nutrition (adapted from Bateson *et al*, 2004)

Conclusion

The recognition that specific mutations may account for some forms of age-related disorder has stimulated much productive research. Certain common polymorphisms (eg apoE) are known to affect susceptibility to age-related disorders and, together with the identification of specific mutations, have facilitated the discovery of biochemical pathways relevant to understanding the genetic determinants of age-related diseases. This approach is not without limitations, however. Recent studies on the contributions of genes to lifespan in lower animals has revealed a family of genes, highly conserved through evolution, that determine lifespan through energy regulation and response to the harmful effects of ageing (inflammation and oxidative stress). Developments such as these indicate the need for testing interventions designed to slow or arrest ageing processes and, potentially, to decrease susceptibility to age-related disease.

Further reading

Andersen SL, Terry DF, Wilcox MA *et al.* Cancer in the oldest old. *Mech Ageing Dev* 2005; **126**: 263–7.

Bateson P, Barker D, Clutton-Brock T *et al.* Developmental plasticity and human health. *Nature* 2004; **430**: 419–21.

Browner WS, Kahn AJ, Ziv E *et al.* The genetics of human longevity. *Am J Med* 2004; **117**: 851–60.

Butler RN, Warner HR, Williams TF *et al.* The aging factor in health and disease: the promise of basic research on aging. *Aging Clin Exp Res* 2004; **16**: 104–11

Christensen H, Mackinnon AJ, Korten A, Jorm AF. The 'common cause hypothesis' of cognitive ageing: evidence for not only a common factor but also specific associations with vision and grip strength in a cross-sectional analysis. *Psychol Aging* 2001; **16**: 588–99.

de Magalhaes JP, Costa J, Toussaint O. HAGR: the Human Ageing Genomic Resources. *Nuc Acid Res* 2005; **33**: Database Issue:D537-43.

Franceschi C, Olivieri F, Marchegiani F *et al.* Genes involved in immune response/inflammation, IGF1/insulin pathway and response to oxidative stress play a major role in the genetics of human longevity: the lesson of centenarians. *Mech Ageing Dev* 2005; **26**: 351–61.

Gambaro G, Anglani F, D'Angelo A. Association studies of genetic polymorphisms and complex diseases. *Lancet* 2000; **355**: 308–11.

Garza AA, Ha TG, Garcia C *et al.* Exercise, antidepressant treatment, and BDNF mRNA expression in the aging brain. *Pharmacol Biochem Behav* 2004; **77**: 209–20.

Longo VD, Finch CE. Genetics of aging and diseases. *Arch Neurol* 2002; **59**: 1706–9.

Martin ER, Lai EH, Gilbert JR *et al.* SNPing away at complex diseases: analysis of a single-nucleotide polymorphisms around APOE in Alzheimer's disease. *Am J Hum Genet* 2000; **67**: 383–94.

Mattson MP, Maudsley S, Martin B. A neural signalling triumvirate that influences ageing and age-related disease: insulin/IGF-1, BDNF and serotonin. *Ageing Research Reviews* 2004; **3**: 445–64.

Mattson MP. Pathways towards and away from Alzheimer's disease. *Nature* 2004; **430**: 631–9.

Miller RA. A position paper on longevity genes. *Sci Aging Knowledge Environ* 2001; **2001(9)**: vp6.

Perls T, Terry D. Genetics of exceptional longevity. *Exp Gerontol* 2003; **38**: 725–30.

Ruse CE, Parker SG. Molecular genetics and age-related disease. *Age Ageing* 2001; **30**: 449–54.

Scott WK, Nance MA, Watts RL *et al.* Complete genomic screen in Parkinson disease – evidence for multiple genes. *JAMA* 2001; **286**: 2239–44.

Terry DF, Wilcox M, McCormick MA *et al.* Cardiovascular advantages among the offspring of centenarians. *J Gerontol A Biol Sci Med Sci* 2003; **58**: M425-31.

Trejo JL, Carro E, Lopez-Lopez C, Torres-Aleman I. Role of serum insulin-like growth factor I in mammalian brain aging. *Growth Horm IGF Res* 2004; **14 (suppl A)**: S3–43.

Whalley LJ. *The Ageing Brain*. London: Orion Books, 2002.

2 Life course risk factors for menopause and diseases in later life

Rebecca Hardy, Gita Mishra and Diana Kuh

Introduction

Life course epidemiology studies the biological and social factors throughout life, including during fetal development, which might act independently, cumulatively or interactively, to influence health and disease later in life. There is growing evidence that women's reproductive characteristics are one component of this risk, either revealing or having a direct influence on latent chronic disease that will become apparent in later life. The following are all associated with later function and disease risk:

- age at menarche
- parity
- conditions during pregnancy
- menstrual or gynaecological disorders
- menopausal vasomotor symptoms
- age at menopause.

Evidence of continuity in reproductive function throughout the life course suggests that lifelong reproductive characteristics may be at least partially determined early in life. Menopause is the most prominent marker of reproductive ageing and has biological and social implications for women's health in midlife and beyond. The age at which a woman reaches the menopause may therefore be both a marker of earlier reproductive health and of later chronic disease status.

A life course approach to chronic disease and ageing

Adult risk factors

A life course approach acknowledges the importance of both genes and the classic adult risk factors to health in later life. Traditionally risk factors and health-related behaviours, such as blood pressure, body composition, cigarette smoking, diet and physical activity, were measured once at baseline and then related to subsequent disease development. In contrast, life course epidemiology examines the effect of these factors at all stages of life. Behaviours track, at least to some extent, between childhood and adult life. So even if it is behaviour in adulthood that has the strongest association with disease risk, interventions to alter lifelong behaviour may be more successful when targeted at children and adolescents. In some instances, such as in the case of cigarette smoking and lung cancer, it will be cumulative exposure that influences disease risk. In others, exposure during a particularly susceptible period of development may be important. For example one study suggested that smoking increased the risk of premenopausal breast cancer only when it occurred within five years of age at menarche.

Biological programming in utero

A life course approach is particularly interested in developmental influences on health and incorporates the concept of 'biological programming'. According to the Barker hypothesis, environmental insults, such as undernutrition during critical periods of fetal growth, have long-term effects on adult disease risk by 'programming' the structure or function of organs, tissues or body systems. The theory is supported by animal experiments and epidemiological observations linking various proxy markers of poor fetal growth, such as low birth weight, with an increased risk of ischaemic heart disease, stroke, diabetes, respiratory disease and their associated adult risk factors such as hypertension and insulin resistance.

The Barker hypothesis has generated much interest and controversy. According to systematic reviews the associations between birth weight and blood pressure and lipid levels are small and are of little public health relevance. Others argue that the importance of fetal growth lies in its influence on disease endpoints, and that the mechanism through which fetal growth has an impact on cardiovascular disease (CVD) is not necessarily through the traditional risk factors. The role of fetal growth in many other aspects of adult health has also been investigated. For example, lighter babies also have poorer muscle strength and cognitive function in adult life. Conversely, breast cancer risk appears to be higher in larger babies, possibly because of a greater exposure to oestrogen *in utero*.

Postnatal growth

The effects of postnatal growth on adult health have recently attracted interest. Rapid increases in body mass index (BMI) during childhood and adolescence have a detrimental impact on cardiovascular health in later life and fast height growth in childhood may increase breast cancer risk. Later body size may also modify the impact of fetal growth. Identifying the critical period of growth is analytically complex and requires longitudinal measures of body size at birth and throughout childhood and adolescence as well as adult height and weight.

Socioeconomic differentials

Low social class in early life has been associated with adverse health outcomes, such as CVD and obesity, and also with poorer adult health-related behaviours (after accounting for adult socioeconomic circumstances). Childhood growth and nutrition are potential factors underlying these associations. Conversely, the associations between birth weight and adult health might be a result of socioeconomic confounding, although this suggestion has so far not been supported by empirical findings. Whatever the relationships between early growth and early socioeconomic conditions are found to be, the underlying biological mechanisms linking the early environment with later health are only just starting to be understood – insulin-like growth factors and inflammation are possible candidates.

Reproductive health from menarche to menopause

Reproductive health is not only integral to women's health and wellbeing but is increasingly recognized as a sentinel of chronic disease in later life. For example, early menarche is associated with breast and ovarian cancers. Women with regular menstrual cycles have lower cardiovascular risk, perhaps reflecting a link between polycystic ovary syndrome and metabolic disturbances characteristic of impaired cardiovascular function. High parity is also associated with CVD risk, probably reflecting the biological stress of pregnancy as well as adverse socioeconomic and lifestyle factors associated with childrearing. Mothers who have offspring of low birth weight are themselves more likely to develop CVD later in life.

Indicators of reproductive ageing are also related to chronic disease risk. Unlike most systems that age slowly and continue to function until death, the loss of reproductive function occurs in middle life. The median age at menopause, the most prominent marker of reproductive ageing, is around 50–52 years in the western industrialized countries, with wide variation between individual women. Early menopause is associated with an increased risk of osteoporosis and late menopause with an increased risk of breast cancer. Both are oestrogen-dependent conditions. Early menopause may also be associated with increased CVD risk and faster cognitive decline, but the evidence is less consistent.

The loss of ovarian follicles throughout intrauterine and postnatal life, even before ovulation begins, supports the relevance of a life course approach to understanding lifelong reproductive function and menopause. The view that the exhaustion of the pool of growing ovarian follicles triggers the menopause has more recently been challenged. Growing evidence suggests that age-related changes to the central nervous system may be the trigger and that the exhaustion of the ovarian follicles is a consequence of the alteration of the neural signal. While estimates of heritability (ranging from 30–70%) from studies of monozygotic and dizygotic twin pairs have indicated that the genetic effect on timing of menopause is considerable, there remains scope for environmental factors to exert an influence.

Life course influences on age at menopause

Cigarette smoking and reproductive characteristics

Of all the adult behavioural and lifestyle factors investigated, only cigarette smoking and nulliparity have consistently been related to an earlier menopause. Through smoking, a cumulative toxic effect on the follicles may lead to faster rates of atresia. However, it has been suggested that oestrogen reduction as a result of smoking may only be critical during the menopausal transition when it amplifies the effect of the naturally decreasing hormone levels. This could also explain the observed shorter perimenopause in smokers compared with non-smokers.

Earlier reproductive characteristics are also associated with timing of menopause. As well as nulliparous women having an earlier menopause than parous women, a later age at menopause has been observed with increasing number of pregnancies. This is consistent with the hypothesis that the fewer ovulatory cycles a woman has throughout her life the later the menopause. However, such an hypothesis is too simplistic and there has been little consistency in findings relating to OC use, history of irregular and long menstrual cycles and later menarche, all of which would also be expected to delay menopause. Alternatively, this finding highlights the potential continuity in a woman's reproductive function where the size of the initial follicle reserve at birth may determine fertility as well as age at menopause. The only study to investigate more specific measures of subfertility and age at menopause found an association between early menopause and:

- miscarriage
- consulting a physician for fertility problems
- having an interval of five or more years between the birth of their first and second child.

Growth and nutrition

Although evidence from mice experiments raises the possibility of postnatal generation of new follicles, the prevailing view has been that a woman is born with an exhaustible and non-renewable supply of ovarian follicles. Little is known about the factors that influence the size of the initial pool of ovarian follicles (although genetics and chance processes will play a role) or about the rate of postnatal follicular atresia prior to the start of ovulation. It is biologically plausible that *in utero* growth and nutrition may be implicated, but two British cohort studies and a twin study found no association between birth weight and age at menopause. Both cohort studies did find that lighter weight in infancy was associated with an earlier menopause. One of these also observed that women who had been bottle fed in infancy as opposed to breastfed had an earlier menopause.

Further evidence that early nutrition or growth might be important comes from a study of women in New Guinea. The median age of menopause in a population who had suffered severe and prolonged malnourishment, and who were of short height and low weight, was estimated to be 4 years earlier than women in the same region with better nourishment. Therefore, malnourishment (possibly acting prenatally through maternal under-nutrition or postnatally through poor childhood growth) may play a role in early menopause. A study of the Dutch famine of 1944–45 points to the importance of postnatal nutrition, as women who had been severely exposed to the famine, especially those who had been aged 2–6 years, had an earlier menopause than unexposed women. The findings relating BMI and weight to age at menopause in well-nourished populations have been mixed, but the impacts of lifetime weight trajectories or lifetime nutrition have hardly been considered.

Socioeconomic status, stress and cognition

Most studies that show any relationship between socioeconomic status in adult life and age at menopause find that the lower the status the earlier the menopause. Few studies have considered socioeconomic status or stress over the life course and age at menopause, even though it may be cumulative stress and hardship experienced throughout the life course that leads to premature ageing of the reproductive system. Bromberger *et al*, having observed that psychosocial stress was associated with early menopause in African–

American women, hypothesized that hypothalamic dysfunction may play a role in the cessation of menses. This is consistent with other evidence of a relationship between the hypothalamic-pituitary-adrenal axis and reproductive function throughout the life course.

In a prospective British birth cohort study, early life socioeconomic status was more strongly associated with age at menopause than adult status. The possibility that early emotional stress may also contribute was raised by the fact that women who experienced parental divorce early in life had an earlier menopause than others. The earlier age at menopause in women from poorer socioeconomic conditions was not due to adult socioeconomic status, behaviour and lifestyle or adult psychological health and stress, but appeared to be partially explained by the early life factors of infant feeding and childhood cognitive ability. A number of studies have now found a link between lower cognitive ability in childhood and adolescence and earlier menopause. Common early environmental or genetic programming of both cognitive and ovarian development may be responsible.

Common risk factors and mechanisms

The research outlined in the previous sections has implications for the interpretation of findings linking timing of menopause with later health outcomes. Changes in body size and cognitive function across the life course, reproductive characteristics from menarche onwards and the combination of lifetime environmental and genetic factors that give rise to such phenotypic expressions are potentially important common antecedents that may account for the associations between age at menopause and chronic disease risk. For example, the fact that cognitive function early in life appears to be related to age at menopause suggests that prior cognitive function must be taken into account when studying the effects of menopause on subsequent cognitive function and its decline. The link between age at menopause and cognition at 65 years in a cohort from Aberdeen, and cognition at 53 years in a national British cohort, could be explained by childhood cognitive function. This points to there being common environmental or genetic factors, possibly operating through long-term or lifelong hormonal mechanisms, which influence both timing of menopause and lifetime cognitive function. More generally, there are potential childhood risk factors for early menopause, such as:

- not having been breastfed
- poor early growth
- poor socioeconomic conditions that are related to poorer adult health, including worse cognitive function.

Exposures at critical periods of the life course, or cumulative exposure to chemicals in the diet or in the environment could also affect hormone levels as well as subsequent disease risk.

In terms of cardiovascular health, women who reach menopause are more likely to smoke and, possibly, be of lower socioeconomic status, both of which are risk factors for CVD. One study using data from the Framingham cohort has also linked premenopausal high blood pressure and poor lipid profile with early menopause, but this has yet to be replicated. Carriers of the factor V Leiden mutation, which is a clotting factor, may also be at higher risk of early menopause, accelerated ageing and CVD. Type I diabetes, a risk factor for early mortality and CVD, has been linked with an earlier age of menopause independent of other known factors. Vascular deterioration, a marker of general ageing as well as CVD risk, is another mechanism through which menopause and later cardiovascular, cognitive and other health outcomes are associated.

Conclusion

The ideas presented here that link reproductive health and chronic disease through common risk factors acting across the life course, relate to what has been termed the 'common cause' approach to ageing. This has been discussed mainly in terms of the relationship between cognitive and physical function and their decline but is obviously relevant to other aspects of adult health and disease risk that change with age. The 'common cause' approach hypothesizes that common endocrine, autonomic and immune mechanisms underlie changes in body size and musculoskeletal, cardiovascular and cognitive function. The evidence suggests the 'common cause' approach needs to consider the extent to which these mechanisms reflect initial developmental differences or common ageing processes.

Further life course studies of the relationships between chronic disease and lifetime reproductive health are warranted to clarify the developmental processes that determine not only age at menopause, but also reproductive health across the life course and risk of chronic disease. The possibility of identifying women at risk of chronic disease through their reproductive health also offers the opportunity of timely and targeted intervention.

Further reading

Barker DJP. *Mothers, babies and health in later life*. Edinburgh: Churchill Livingstone, 1998.

Bromberger JT, Matthews KA, Kuller LH *et al.* Prospective study of the determinants of age at menopause. *Am J Epidemiol* 1997; **145**: 124–33.

Christensen H, Mackinnon AJ, Korten A, Jorm AF. The 'common cause hypothesis' of cognitive aging: evidence for not only a common factor but also specific associations of age with vision and grip strength in a cross-sectional analysis. *Psychol Aging* 2001; **16**: 588–99.

Cresswell JL, Egger P, Fall CHD *et al.* Is the age of menopause determined in-utero? *Early Hum Dev* 1997; **49**: 143–8.

Dorman JS, Steenkiste AR, Foley TP *et al.* Menopause in type 1 diabetic women: is it premature? *Diabetes* 2001; **50**: 1857–62.

Elias SG, van Noord PAH, Peeters PHM *et al.* Caloric restriction reduces age at menopause: the effect of the 1944–1945 Dutch famine. *Menopause* 2003; **10**: 399–405.

Finch CE, Kirkwood TBL. *Chance, Development and Aging.* Oxford: Oxford University Press, 2000.

Hardy R, Kuh D. Menopause and gynaecological disorders: a life course perspective. In: Kuh, D, Hardy, R (Eds). *A life course approach to women's health.* Oxford University Press: Oxford, 2002: 64–85.

Hardy R, Kuh D. Does early growth influence timing of the menopause? Evidence from a British birth cohort. *Hum Reprod* 2002; **17**: 2474–9.

Hardy R, Kuh D. Social and environmental conditions across the life course and age at menopause in a British birth cohort study. *Br J Obstet Gynaecol* 2005; **112**: 346–54.

Huxley R, Neil A, Collins R. Unravelling the fetal origins hypothesis: is there really an inverse association between birthweight and subsequent blood pressure? *Lancet* 2002; **360**: 659–65.

Johnson J, Canning J, Kaneko T *et al.* Germline stem cells and follicular renewal in the postnatal mammalian ovary. *Nature* 2004; **428**: 145–50.

Kok HS, van Asselt KM, van der Schouw YT *et al.* Subfertility reflects accelerated ovarian ageing. *Hum Reprod* 2003; **18**: 644–8.

Kok HS, Kuh D, Cooper R *et al.* Cognitive function across the life course and the menopausal transition in a British birth cohort. *Menopause* 2005. In press.

Kuh D, Ben-Shlomo Y. *A life course approach to chronic disease epidemiology (2nd edition).* Oxford: Oxford University Press, 2004.

Kuh D, Butterworth S, Kok H *et al.* Childhood cognitive ability and age at menopause: evidence from two cohort studies. *Menopause* 2005. In press.

Owen CG, Whincup PH, Odoki K *et al.* Birth weight and blood cholesterol level: a study in adolescents and systematic review. *Pediatrics* 2003; **111**: 1081–9.

Rich-Edwards J. A life course approach to women's reproductive health. In: Kuh D, Hardy R (Eds). *A life course approach to women's health.* Oxford University Press: Oxford, 2002; pp 23–43.

Rich-Edwards JW, Kleinman K, Michels KB *et al.* Longitudinal study of birth weight and adult body mass index in predicting risk of coronary heart disease and stroke in women. *BMJ* 2005; Epub 27 April 2005.

Scragg RFR. *Menopause and reproductive span in rural Niugini. Proceedings of the annual symposium of the Papua New Guinea Medical Society.* Papua New Guinea Medical Society: Port Moresby, 1973; pp 126–44.

Treloar SA, Sadrzadeh S, Do K-A *et al.* Birth weight and age at menopause in Australian female twin pairs: exploration of the fetal origin hypothesis. *Hum Reprod* 2000; **15**: 55–9.

van Asselt KM, Kok HS, Peeters PHM *et al.* Factor V Leiden mutation accelerates the onset of natural menopause. *Menopause* 2003; **10**: 477–81.

van Asselt KM, Kok HS, van der Schouw YT *et al.* Current smoking at menopause rather than duration determines the onset of natural menopause. *Epidemiology* 2004; **15**: 634–9.

Whalley LJ, Fox HC, Starr JM, Deary IJ. Age at natural menopause and cognition. *Maturitas* 2004; **49**: 148–56.

Wise PM, Krajnak KM, Kashon ML. Menopause: the aging of multiple pacemakers. *Science* 1996; **273**: 67–70.

3 Dementia

Bob Barber, Sarah Daley and John O'Brien

Introduction

Dementia is a chronic illness affecting many central human characteristics, the most important of which include:

- memory and cognition
- behaviour
- personality traits
- level of independence
- physical and neurological function.

In dementia there is a chronic impairment of cognitive faculties. There are also prominent changes in behaviour and personality, and a person's physical and neurological status will ultimately deteriorate.

A wide variety of disorders can cause dementia, and these are summarized in Table 3.1. In general, individual diseases have distinct clinical presentations because they affect specific areas of the brain in different ways. Depending on the underlying pathology, the illness may be reversible, static or most commonly progressive.

Dementia is analogous to the syndrome of 'chronic brain failure'. In contrast, delirium refers to the syndrome of 'acute brain failure', which, unlike dementia, is associated with reduced attention or consciousness. Importantly, because a person with dementia may have pre-existing brain disease, they are at a greater risk of developing delirium. When these syndromes co-exist, as they often do, the interaction leads to an 'acute-on-chronic' deterioration.

Table 3.1
Causes of dementia

Category	Examples of Disorders
Degenerative	Alzheimer's disease Dementia with Lewy bodies Frontotemporal dementia Progressive supranuclear palsy Multi-system atrophy
Vascular	Cerebrovascular disease* Hypoperfusion (eg after cardiac arrest or septicaemia)* Chronic subdural haematoma* Rare: CADASIL (cerebral autosomal dominant arteriopathy with subcortical infarcts and leukoencephalopathy) Vasculitis*
Alcohol/toxic/drug	Alcohol related*, includes alcohol-related dementia; Wernicke-Korsakoff syndrome
Infective and prion-related	Prion disorders (eg Creutzfeldt-Jacob disease) Syphilis* Encephalitis* HIV-related*
Traumatic	Head injuries
Endocrine & metabolic disorders	Hypo/hyperthyroid disease* Wilson's disease*
Nutritional	Vitamin deficiencies* (vitamin B12, folic acid, thiamine)
Genetic	Huntington's disease
Neoplasm	Primary* or secondary central nervous system tumours
Hydrocephalus	Normal pressure hydrocephalus*
Demylinating disorders	Multiple sclerosis (as a late complication)

* treating the underlying cause can potentially modify the course

Extent of the problem

Dementia is a common but not inevitable consequence of ageing. Its prevalence and incidence increases with age and the risk of developing dementia doubles every five years after age 65. Approximately 7% of people aged over 65 years are affected, increasing to at least 20% in people aged 80 years and over. It may exceed 50% in those over 90.

In the UK, there are an estimated 750 000 people with dementia and this includes over 18 000 people aged under 65 years. In the USA there are 4–5 million sufferers, and 25 million worldwide. The prevalence and incidence of dementia shows little geographical variation, but worldwide the majority of patients with dementia live in less developed regions. As more people are living longer, the total number of people affected will continue to increase, with an estimated 1.8 million affected in the UK by 2050 and 114 million worldwide.

Impact of dementia

The average life expectancy of a person with dementia is 3–7 years after the diagnosis is made, although diagnosis often occurs some years after first onset of symptoms. It is the fourth most common cause of death after heart disease, cancer and stroke. The World Health Organization recognizes dementia as one of the major causes of disability worldwide. It causes significant distress to patients, their carers and families and has an enormous impact on society. In England alone, the total cost of dementia care ('formal' and 'informal') is calculated to be £6.1 billion (US$11.6 billion, Euro 8.8 billion) (1998/99 prices), with £3.3 billion (US$6.31 billion, Euro 4.78 billion) of this total being direct spending by health and social services. Most people with dementia live in the community and require a range of supportive services, and in the long term they are likely to require residential or nursing home care. Indeed, an estimated 50% of all nursing home residents suffer from dementia (see Chapter 10). Dementia also has an adverse impact on a range of outcomes in acute hospital settings, including:

- an increase in mortality
- increased length of stay
- increased likelihood of institutionalization.

Table 3.2 summarizes some of the main direct and indirect consequences of the illness for women. It is important to stress that although cognitive impairment is a central feature of dementia, psychological and behavioural changes are also common and important symptoms. These frequently cause carer stress and are major factors leading to hospital admission and/or institutional care. Women have a central role in providing care and support to people with dementia, either as a member of a family or as a voluntary or aid carer.

Common forms of dementia in late life

The three commonest causes of dementia are summarized below and in Table 3.3.

Table 3.2
Impact on women

Women as...	Direct
Patients	Distress and symptoms of illness Effects upon role as spouse/carer/sibling/parent Changes within the home/family Increased dependency on others Decreased independence (eg driving) Move into institutional care (financial implications) Complications of treatments used for symptom management (eg falls, fractures, hyperprolactinaemia, osteoporosis, cerebrovascular disease)
Carers	Imposes significant burden Risks to mental health (particularly depression) and physical health (eg due to physical interventions, such as lifting/moving) As a carer, social isolation, fear/uncertainty, loneliness – loss of intimacy/reciprocity, grieving, stigmatization, disruption of family life, decreased quality of life, financial loss
Members of society	Women are more likely to be both formal and informal carers High costs to society generally

Alzheimer's disease

Alzheimer's disease (AD) is the most common cause of dementia in older people, and accounts for 50–60% of all dementia sufferers. It is more common in women, particularly in those aged over 80 years (ratio 1.5:1). The female predominance is due to both an increase in prevalence, partly as women live longer, and also an increase in incidence. Characteristically, a person experiences a gradual decline in cognitive function, with core changes summarized as:

- amnesia (memory)
- apraxia (action)
- agnosia (recognition)
- aphasia (spoken language)
- alexia (reading)
- agraphia (writing)
- acalculia (calculation).

Table 3.3

Clinical features of the main causes of dementia

	Alzheimer's disease	**Vascular dementia**	**Dementia with Lewy bodies**
Course	Progressive	Abrupt onset Stepwise related to infarcts, although small vessel disease progression is more gradual	Fluctuating cognitive performance and conscious level
Pattern of cognitive decline	Amnesia: recent memories before remote Apraxia: impairments with motor tasks, eg dressing Agnosia: difficulties with object recognition and naming Aphasia: word finding and communication difficulties	Memory deficits less severe than with AD Slowed thinking Impaired executive functioning Nocturnal confusion	Impaired attention and alertness Prominent visuospatial deficits (>memory loss)
Behavioural and psychological symptoms of dementia	Delusions/visual hallucinations in later stages Depression Agitation Wandering Sleep disturbance Apathy	Delusions/visual hallucinations in later stages Depression (VaD>AD) Emotional lability Anxiety Agitation Irritability Apathy	Visual hallucinations common (+/- delusions), especially early Depression

Table 3.3 continued

	Alzheimer's disease	Vascular dementia	Dementia with Lewy bodies
Salient features on examination	Nothing specific	Focal signs Sensory/motor deficits Gait disturbance Unsteadiness/unprovoked falls	Rigidity Bradykinesia Parkinsonian gait Postural hypotension Repeated falls
Neuroimaging CT/MRI	Generalized atrophy (especially medial temporal lobes) Ventricular enlargement Less white matter change than VaD but similar to DLB	Generalized atrophy Ventricular enlargement Infarcts and/or significant white matter change	Generalized atrophy (relative sparing of medial temporal lobe structures) Ventricular enlargement
SPECT	Global ↓ perfusion but especially bilateral temporal–parietal	Patchy deficits	Global ↓ (especially occipital)

MRI, magnetic resonance imaging; CT, computer tomography; SPECT, single photon emission computer tomography; AD, Alzheimer's disease; VaD, vascular dementia; DLB, dementia with Lewy bodies

Visuospatial deficits are also very common and, coupled with failing short-term memory, they lead to disorientation in time and eventually place. Psychological and behavioural changes include irritability, agitation, apathy, depression and psychosis.

Vascular dementia

Vascular dementia (VaD) is the second most common cause of dementia, accounting for about 20% of late-life dementia. It is relatively more common in men than women, especially in men under 75 years of age. The symptoms experienced will in part be determined by the extent and localization of cerebrovascular disease. As with AD, psychological and behavioural changes are common.

Dementia with Lewy bodies

The third most frequent cause of dementia in late life is dementia with Lewy bodies (DLB), which occurs in about 10–15% of people. It primarily affects people over the age of 70 years and is slightly more common in men. The core clinical features of this disorder are the triad of fluctuating cognitive impairment, persistent visual hallucinations and spontaneous parkinsonism. In practice, DLB is under-diagnosed but is clinically important because the management of the symptoms can be complex and, at times, hazardous. Patients can be exquisitely sensitive to antipsychotic medication and the use of these medications should be avoided. Specialist referral is often necessary.

Pathology

Alzheimer's disease

The precise causal pathway in AD is not known but the main theory focuses on the abnormal build up of two proteins in and around neurons. These are intracellular hyperphosphorylated tau (in neurofibrillary 'tangles') and extracellular amyloid (in senile 'plaques'). Abnormalities in the synthesis and/or clearance of these proteins are hypothesized to lead to cell dysfunction and eventual cell death, which can be visualized in life as atrophy on brain imaging. These changes first develop in the memory centres of the brain a number of years before the onset of symptoms. Intriguingly AD shares some common risk factors with VaD, as outlined in Table 3.4

AD is associated with a loss of cholinergic function, notably acetylcholine (ACh). This is a key neurotransmitter involved in memory and attention, as well as symptoms like hallucinations. Cholinesterase inhibitors are the main

Table 3.4
Risk factors for main causes of dementia

	Main Risk Factors	Comments
AD	Age Family History Female gender Genetic mutations (in early onset dementia) Down's Syndrome Depression (perhaps mediated by increased stress and cortisol levels) Low education (better education may reflect greater cognitive capacity and reserve, thereby deferring the onset of the illness.) Repetitive head injuries Vascular risk factors (insulin-dependent diabetes, hypertension and raised cholesterol)	Vascular risk factors have been associated with increase in AD as well as VaD Cognitive and leisure activity may be protective, as might light-to-moderate consumption of wine Various dietary factors have been suggested as beneficial in preventing AD but evidence is not conclusive: these include – vitamins (folate, Vit B6 & Vit B12), unsaturated fatty acids, and fish oil (omega-3 polyunsaturated fatty acids)
VaD	Age Male gender Vascular risk factors for stroke, eg hypertension, diabetes, heart disease (atrial fibrillation, valvular and ischaemic disease), raised cholesterol, smoking Family history Polycythaemia	More potentially modifiable risk factors
DLB	Male gender Parkinson's disease Genetic abnormality involving alpha-synuclein	

AD, Alzheimer's disease; VaD, vascular dementia; DLB, dementia with Lewy bodies

pharmacological treatments in AD, and act by inhibiting the enzyme acetylcholinesterase, which degrades ACh.

Vascular dementia

VaD is pathologically heterogeneous and there is no single signature of symptoms. Subtypes of VaD include multi-infarct dementia, strategic single infarct dementia and small vessel disease with dementia, although other mechanisms can also exist. In contrast to AD, where available treatments focus on symptom management, the standard interventions for VaD aim to modify disease progression by optimizing management of any vascular risk factors, as for stroke disease.

Dementia with Lewy bodies

A spectrum of Lewy body disorders exists with the clinical features reflecting the distribution of pathology. In Parkinson's disease (PD) 'Lewy bodies' (LB) in the brain stem are prominent and they are associated with the motor symptoms of PD. In DLB, LB are more widely distributed in the limbic and neocortical regions and are implicated in the cognitive and neuropsychiatric symptoms. LB can also occur in the spinal cord sympathetic neurons and dorsal vagal nuclei leading to autonomic failure and dysphagia, respectively. Although 'pure' presentations are seen, heterogeneous combinations of parkinsonism, cognitive impairment, neuropsychiatric symptoms and signs of autonomic failure reflecting multi-site (diffuse) pathology are more frequent, especially in the elderly. Neurochemical changes also feature prominently, particularly deficits in ACh and dopamine. As with AD, the deficits in ACh form the rationale for using cholinesterase inhibitors in DLB.

Role of oestrogens

The observation that postmenopausal women are more likely to develop Alzheimer's disease than men has naturally lead to speculation that oestrogen deficiency associated with menopause may contribute to the development of AD, perhaps by inducing a state of accelerated ageing. The practical implication of this 'oestrogen deficiency (or neuroprotective) hypothesis' of dementia is to suggest that oestrogen replacement therapy would be useful for preventing or delaying the onset of this dementia, and could potentially benefit patients with established AD.

But what is the evidence that oestrogen can have beneficial effects on brain structures? Suggested mechanisms include protection against:

- amyloid formation
- oxidative stress
- vascular disease
- neuronal loss
- loss of cholinergic transmission.

However, findings from clinical studies have been mixed, with both positive and negative results.

Box 3.1

Practical guide to the assessment and management of dementia

Step 1: Initial detection and benefits of early diagnosis
The diagnosis of dementia is clinically based. There are no biological diagnostic markers, although certain investigations can improve diagnostic confidence. Family members have a crucial role in establishing an accurate clinical history and usually initiate the first contact with a family physician. Timely and accurate diagnosis allows for early intervention and greater planning for the future.

The aim of any examination and investigation is at least two-fold. First – to clarify the specific diagnosis and exclude other potential causes, such as delirium or depression. Second – when a dementia is present, it is important to detect any co-morbid factors that could influence treatment options (such as cardiac arrhythmias, impaired renal or liver function) and/or exacerbate symptoms of the illness (such as anaemia, infections, cardiac failure, pain). Table 3.5 outlines some initial steps in the medical assessment of dementia.

Step 2: Providing information
Explaining the diagnosis and providing information to individuals and their families is an important but potentially sensitive and difficult area. The Alzheimer's Society in the UK (www.alzheimers.org.uk) and the USA-based Alzheimer's Association (www.alz.org) are a useful source of help and information.

Step 3. Establishing the key issues to target interventions and planning further assessments
The clinician will need to work with other professionals and agencies hand-in-hand with the patient and their family. Input may be sought in the form of occupational therapy, environmental adaptations and mobility aids, social worker and community supports, financial and legal advice, physiotherapy, and community psychiatric nurses as appropriate.

Consideration will need to be given to a range of issues including level of psychiatric symptoms, functioning, safety, risks, mobility, medication compliance and driving, as well as physical health, environmental, social, personal and nutritional needs. Expectations and wishes of the patient and their family need to be clarified as do the strains and strengths of the care network.

Step 4. Initial management: the importance of non-pharmacological approaches
Although systematic evidence of psychosocial interventions in dementia is limited, the provision of educational, practical and emotional support for patients and carers will form the backbone of clinical management. Patients may also benefit from certain interventions, such as reality reorientation.

Step 5: Referral to a specialist and pharmacological management
Reasons to refer to a specialist include diagnostic uncertainties, access to specific treatments or interventions, and when there are concerns about safety, risks, level of psychiatric disturbance or carer stress.

Table 3.5
Initial medical assessments in dementia

Physical examination:	At least cardiovascular and neurological systems – although tailored to the specific differential diagnosis
Mental state examination	Assess presence and severity of any psychiatric and cognitive symptoms Standardized screening tool, such as the mini-mental state examination (MMSE) is a useful way to detect deficits (and areas of preserved functioning) Clock drawing test can quickly and usefully reveal signs of dyspraxia
Investigations	Standard 'dementia screen', eg full blood count, erythrocyte sedimentation rate, urea and electrolytes, liver function, thyroid function, vitamin B12 and folate, and cholesterol Appropriate consideration should be given to further investigations as relevant, eg electrocardiogram, chest x-ray and urine analysis

The most important recent findings have come from the USA multi-centre Women's Health Initiative Memory Study (WHIMS). The study aimed to evaluate the effects of treatment with oestrogen and oestrogen plus progestogen in postmenopausal women over 65 years of age on the incidence of dementia and mild cognitive impairment (MCI). The oestrogen plus progestogen arm of the trial was discontinued in 2002 and the oestrogen-alone arm in 2004. In both arms participants receiving active treatment were twice as likely to develop dementia compared with placebo. The increased risk was seen in AD and VaD. In addition, there was no beneficial effect on the incidence of mild cognitive impairment and treatment had no positive impact on measures of cognitive function – indeed there was a small increased risk of clinically meaningful decline in the active treatment group.

In terms of treatment of established AD, initially encouraging findings have not been confirmed by more recent randomized clinical trials. Conjugated equine oestrogens, alone and in combination with a progestogen, have shown no benefit for the treatment of established AD and the Cochrane systematic review on this topic also concluded that hormone replacement therapy (HRT) or oestrogen replacement therapy for cognitive improvement or maintenance is not indicated for women with AD.

In summary, based on current evidence, there is presently no role for oestrogen replacement therapy in the treatment or prevention of AD or cognitive decline. However, it is still conceivable that any potential neuroprotective role of HRT could occur at the very initial, preclinical stages of pathology with a so-called ' window of opportunity', but once established, HRT has little if any impact.

Pharmacological treatment

As summarized in Table 3.6, the main pharmacological treatment options are cholinesterase inhibitors, memantine, antipsychotics and antidepressants.

Cholinesterase inhibitors (donepezil, galantamine and rivastigmine) are increasingly viewed as first-line treatment in mild-to-moderate AD. Compared to placebo, efficacy has been established in terms of cognitive improvement and activities of daily living. They also improve psychiatric symptoms, such as psychosis and apathy, in both AD and DLB. Currently, the three drugs are thought to have similar efficacy but differ in terms of dosing regime, side-effect profile and drug interactions. In the first year or so of treatment, the mean effect is equivalent to an improvement in cognition that is comparable to 6–9 months of naturalistic decline, although there is a marked heterogeneity of response, with some patients responding with a clear improvement and others not responding at all. After one year, cognitive performance will usually decline but remain higher than that estimated for untreated patients. Long-term benefits might include delayed admission into 24-hour care.

There are no reliable predictors of response, nor any evidence that the drugs have a disease-modifying effect. Common side-effects include:

- nausea and vomiting
- loss of appetite
- diarrhoea
- headaches
- dizziness.

Occasionally increased agitation and irritability can occur and caution is required in certain patients with cardiac conduction abnormalities, particularly those with bradycardia. Specialists prescribe the drugs and they are usually initiated on a trial basis for 4–6 months to establish whether the intervention has been beneficial; if not, then treatment is usually withdrawn.

Memantine was approved in 2002 by the European Agency for the Evaluation of Medical Products and in 2003 by the USA Federal Drug Administration for the treatment of moderately-severe to severe AD. It is an uncompetitive N-methyl-D-aspartate (NMDA) receptor antagonist that is

Table 3.6

Drug interventions in dementia

Class	Examples	Common uses	Comments
Cholinesterase inhibitors	Donepezil Galantamine Rivastigmine	Mild to moderate AD (and DLB) for symptomatic management of cognitive and non-cognitive symptoms (Also off-license use by specialists in DLB)	Started under specialist advice usually on a trial basis to assess efficacy and tolerability
N-methyl-D-aspartate (NMDA) receptor antagonist	Memantine	Moderate to severe AD	Used under specialist advice. Patients may deteriorate less slowly; usually reserved for people with advanced dementia who are living at home
Antidepressants	Serotonin-selective re-uptake inhibitors (SSRIs)	Depressive symptoms Emotional lability	Avoid tricylic antidepressants because of side-effects, eg falls Emotional lability may respond in days
Antipsychotics	Atypical (eg risperidone 0.5–1mg/day), conventional (haloperidol 0.5–1mg/day)	Psychotic symptoms Severe agitation/aggression	Risperidone and olanzapine are associated with increase risk of cerebrovascular accidents Haloperidol can cause significant extra-pyramidal side-effects All antipsychotics should be avoided in DLB
Clomethiazole	Clomethiazole	Sleep disturbance	Use selectively and on short-term basis
Benzodiazepine	Clonazepam	Myoclonic jerks	
Trazodone	Low-dose trazodone	Sleep disturbance, agitation	
Cardiovascular medications		To manage vascular risk factors	Important intervention for VaD

AD, Alzheimer's disease; VaD, vascular dementia; DLB, dementia with Lewy bodies thought to protect nerve cells from toxic effects of the excitatory neuro-transmitter glutamate. Patients treated with memantine experience less of a decline compared to placebo, rather than an improvement. A recent Cochrane Review concluded that memantine had a positive effect (ie less deterioration) on cognition, mood and behaviour and the ability to perform activities of daily living in patients with moderate to severe AD. Patients were also less likely to become agitated. Its use is usually limited to people living at home with advanced AD under specialist care. It is generally well tolerated and the incidence of adverse effects is low.

Conclusion

Dementia has a profound effect on women, be it through the direct experience of the illness or by virtue of their role as either informal or formal caregivers. Where possible, interventions try to optimize choice and autonomy, but inevitably the provision of support and treatment will need to reflect the progressive and multifaceted nature of the illness. In terms of pharmacological intervention, symptomatic treatments are currently available, but it is now doubtful that oestrogen replacement will have a role in the management of dementia.

Further reading

Areosa Sastre A, McShane R, Sherriff F. Memantine for dementia. *The Cochrane Database of Systematic Reviews* 2004, Issue 4.

Espeland MA, Rapp SR, Shumaker SA *et al.* Conjugated equine estrogens and global cognitive function in postmenopausal women: Women's Health Initiative Memory Study. *JAMA* 2004; **291**: 2959–68.

Hogervorst E, Yaffe K, Richards M, Huppert F. Hormone replacement therapy to maintain cognitive function in women with dementia. *The Cochrane Database of Systematic Reviews* 2002, Issue 3.

Mulnard RA, Corrada MM, Kawas CH. Estrogen replacement therapy, Alzheimer's disease, and mild cognitive impairment. *Curr Neurol Neurosci Rep* 2004; **4**: 368–73.

Rapp SR, Espeland MA, Shumaker SA *et al.* Effect of estrogen plus progestin on global cognitive function in postmenopausal women: the Women's Health Initiative Memory Study: a randomized controlled trial. *JAMA* 2003; **289**: 2663–72.

Shumaker SA, Legault C, Kuller L *et al.* Conjugated equine estrogens and incidence of probable dementia and mild cognitive impairment in postmenopausal women: Women's Health Initiative Memory Study. *JAMA* 2004; **291**: 2947–58.

Shumaker SA, Legault C, Thal L *et al.* Estrogen plus progestin and the incidence of dementia and mild cognitive impairment in postmenopausal women: the Women's Health Initiative Memory Study: a randomized controlled trial. *JAMA* 2003; **289**: 2651–62.

Wimo A, Winblad B, Aguero-Torres H, von Strauss E. The magnitude of dementia occurrence in the world. *Alzheimer Dis Assoc Disord* 2003; **17**: 63–7.

Zandi PP, Carlson MC, Plassman BL *et al.* Hormone replacement therapy and incidence of Alzheimer disease in older women: the Cache County Study. *JAMA* 2002; **288**: 2123–9.

4 Myocardial infarction in women

Wasing Taggu and Guy W L Lloyd

Introduction

Cardiovascular diseases (coronary artery disease and stroke) are the biggest single cause of death among women in both the UK (Figure 4.1) and the western world. Each year in the USA more than half a million women die of cardiovascular (CV) disease, translating into approximately one death every minute. This situation is likely to continue with an ageing population and increasing levels of obesity and diabetes. Despite this, the misconception that

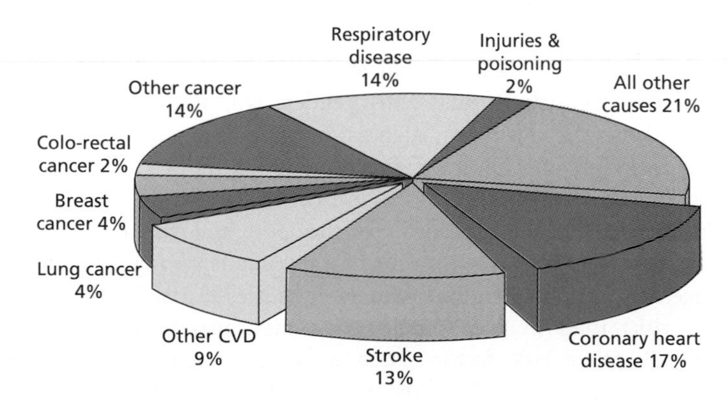

Figure 4.1 Deaths by cause, women, 2002, United Kingdom

coronary artery disease (CAD) primarily affects men and carries a more benign prognosis in women, is an opinion shared, until recently, by both patients and healthcare professionals. This has resulted in a lack of all aspects of cardiovascular prevention, diagnosis and treatment being given to women.

Despite the importance of coronary artery disease in women there are certain key differences from men. The diagnosis appears more difficult for several reasons. Chest pain may not accurately predict the presence of coronary artery disease. Cardiac risk factors, including age, family history, smoking, hypertension, lipoproteins and diabetes are all associated with increased cardiac risk in both genders, but additional factors (in particular endogenous and exogenous female sex hormones) may be important. Most notably, women tend to be 8–10 years older than men at presentation – a factor that may influence both responses to treatment and therapeutic decisions.

Risk factors for myocardial infarction in women

Biological risk factors

Lipid profiles

The lipid profiles of both sexes presenting with myocardial infarction show a similar relationship with cardiac risk. Low-density lipoprotein (LDL)-cholesterol shows a strong positive correlation with increasing cardiac risk while high-density lipoprotein (HDL)-cholesterol is broadly protective. The modulation of LDL-cholesterol (and apoliprotein B-containing particles) using lipid-lowering agents results in some degree of angiographic regression in coronary arteries, but more importantly a reduction in cardiac end-points comparable to that observed with men. During long-term intervention with pravastatin, data from a number of pooled placebo-controlled studies show that men and women shared a similar reduction in cardiac events (23% and 27%, respectively). Although few other statin trials have presented gender-specific outcomes, there is no reason to suspect that the clinical effects of LDL-cholesterol reduction vary with gender. No outcome data are yet available with newer treatments, such as dietary stanol supplementation or ezetimibe, although lipid-lowering efficacy is similar in men and women.

The menopause and sex hormone use have a profound effect on both HDL-cholesterol and triglycerides, so the potential for gender-specific variations in risk associated with these parameters is strong. Meta-analyses have suggested that raised triglycerides confer a greater risk in women (76% increased risk) than in men (32%). This may also be associated with clustering of other risk factors such as central obesity, hypertension, procoagulant states and insulin resistance. Atherogenic remnant lipoprotein fractions consisting of very low-density lipoprotein (VLDL), intermediate-density lipoprotein (IDL) and chylomicron remnants are all associated with high triglyceride levels, as is the predominance of small dense LDL particles, which are strongly atherogenic.

Hypertension

Hypertension carries an independent coronary risk for both sexes, which is multiplicative with the risk associated with smoking, obesity and diabetes. Antihypertensive treatment reduces mortality and morbidity as well as stroke. These effects are most striking in the elderly, a population in which women are generally over-represented.

Smoking

As with men, smoking remains one of the major causal factors of myocardial infarction. The past 30 years have seen major declines in smoking rates among all sectors of society. Young women have shown proportionately the lowest decline, perhaps because of social pressure to maintain weight control (Figure 4.2). This may represent a significant, and as yet underappreciated, future health hazard. Even minimal exposure (five cigarettes/day) constitutes a risk and this is not improved by use of low-yield cigarettes. In women above the age of 35, smoking increases the chance of early menopause, which may accelerate atherogenesis. The combination of smoking and the oral contraceptive pill appears to convey a very high additional risk. This excess risk amongst smokers is of the order of 400 additional infarctions per 1 000 000 treatment years.

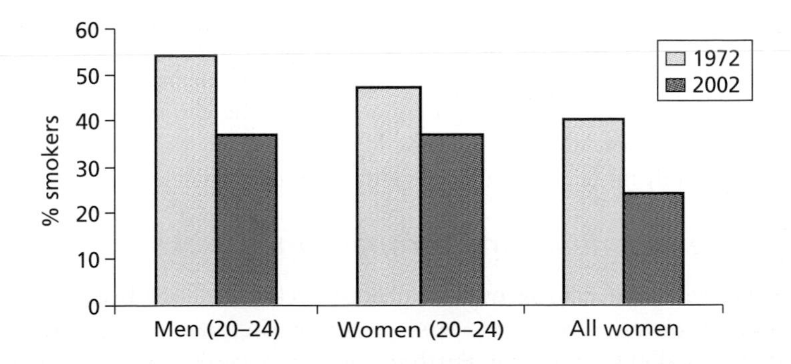

Figure 4.2 Percentage of smokers in younger women and men, as well as all women comparing 1972 with 2002

Exercise

The beneficial effects of exercise on cardiovascular risk factors may be less marked in women compared to men due to a lower absolute weight reduction and a lesser increase in HDL. The Nurses Health Study showed that among women brisk walking could yield similar benefits to vigorous exercise, and that sedentary women who became active late in life reaped similar benefits as those who remained active throughout. Body mass index, waist circumference, waist:hip ratio, and waist:height ratio do not seem to be independently associated with angiographic CAD or adverse CV events.

Chronic inflammation

The presence of a chronic inflammatory response, as characterized by a low-grade increase in high sensitivity C-reactive protein (CRP), is associated with increased risk of myocardial infarction. The reason for this is obscure but it is possible that CRP interacts with lipoproteins to promote atherosclerosis. The nested case-control Women's Health Study of 28 263 women showed that CRP was as powerful an independent predictor as any other single factor. Women with the highest quartile of CRP had a 5–7-fold increased risk of cardiac and vascular events over a three-year follow-up period. Most forms of exogenous female sex hormones appear to increase CRP, which may explain the lack of benefit from these agents as demonstrated in randomized controlled trials.

Psychosocial risk factors

Several of the cardiovascular risk factors discussed above are primarily related to lifestyle choices and are optimally treated by behaviour modification. Acute and chronic stress is thought to trigger myocardial infarction in both sexes by contributing to plaque rupture. Depression appears to be an independent risk factor for poor outcome after acute cardiac events or surgery in women. Limited data suggest that the use of antidepressants after myocardial infarction may reduce overall mortality. Animal models also give insights into the role of society in modulating cardiac risk. In the cymologous monkey model of atherosclerosis, animals at the lower end of the social hierarchy had both appreciably more atherosclerosis and lower oestrogen levels.

Female sex hormones and coronary artery disease

The hypothesis that oestrogens are cardioprotective has long been accepted because coronary disease is less common in women (particularly premenopausally) than in men. Furthermore, oestrogen has a broad range of effects on the atherogenic milieu, many of which should reduce cardiac risk. The final pillar of the hypothesis is that women who take hormone replacement therapy (HRT) are significantly less likely to develop coronary disease than those who do not. Recent evidence from well-designed randomized trials has severely questioned this hypothesis and has even pointed to a potential harmful effect.

There are several flaws in the original hypothesis. While premenopausal women are less likely to have coronary artery disease, there are many confounding factors, in particular the effect of social class and smoking, which influence both coronary risk and menopausal age. The increase of coronary disease in women from age 20 to 75 shows a clear exponential relationship, which is not disturbed by transition through the menopause. If this is compared with breast cancer (a prototype oestrogen-sensitive disease) there is a clear difference with a slackening off of the rate of rise in the incidence of breast cancer at or around the menopause (Figure 4.3). Some data in premenopausal women have suggested that low-oestrogen parts of the menstrual cycle are associated with both angina and myocardial infarction. The effect of surgical menopause on heart disease risk has also been striking so it may be that very rapid loss of oestrogen is one factor that might promote myocardial infarction.

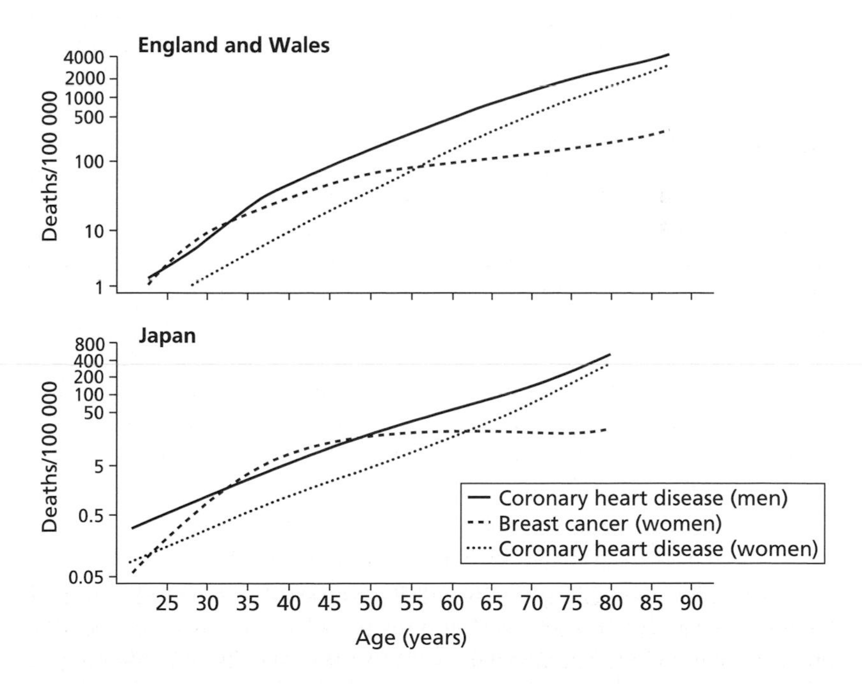

Figure 4.3 Death rates by age and diagnosis form women and men in the UK and Japan
Reproduced with permission from Lawlor D, Ebrahim S, Davey G. *BMJ* 2002; **325**: 311–12

Sex hormones have profound effects on the lipid profile – indeed this has been one of the mainstays of the oestrogen cardioprevention hypothesis. Unfortunately the effect of various different hormone regimes has diverse effects. In particular, the more oestrogenic a compound is, the more likely it is to increase triglycerides and HDL-cholesterol. However, more androgenic compounds, such as tibolone, will tend to have the opposite effect. In general transdermal oestrogen has the least effect on the lipid profile.

In the PEPI study conjugated equine oestrogen (CEE) reduced total cholesterol by 8%, LDL-cholesterol fell by around 15% and HDL-cholesterol increased by between 4–5%, triglycerides also increased. The beneficial effect of CEE on HDL-cholesterol was abolished by the addition of medroxy-progesterone acetate. Oral oestrogen with or without a progestogen reduced lipoprotein-a by between 17–23% at 36 months.

While much attention has focused on the beneficial effects of oestrogen on cardiac risk factors, there are certain detrimental effects. In particular the rise in triglycerides may negate any beneficial effects on LDL-cholesterol by reducing LDL particle size and hence increasing its atherogenicity. Furthermore, most forms of HRT now appear to increase plasma CRP, thus increasing the risk of infarction. The clear increase in venous thrombo-embolic risk associated with HRT, possibly in response to elevations of antithrombin III, might also suggest an increased risk in arterial thrombosis.

The final problem with the oestrogen hypothesis is the difference between the observational evidence, which is almost exclusively favourable, and the randomized evidence, which shows no benefit. Part of the explanation is that women who opt for HRT tend to be at considerably lower cardiac risk, even premenopausally.

The results from a number of randomized trials in various contexts and using a number of different drugs are available. Over 32 000 subjects have been studied for between 3–8 years (Table 4.1). None of these randomized studies has shown a significant beneficial effect of the drugs. This is as true for both opposed and unopposed oestrogen as it is for conjugated oestrogens compared with 17-β-oestradiol. Furthermore, transdermal oestrogen seems to have a similar negative effect. Many of the studies have suggested the possibility of a small increased risk of myocardial infarction of the order of 27%, which is maximal in the year after treatment initiation. Most of the randomized data suggest that HRT increases the risk of stroke. No long-term randomized data are available for tibolone, although its differential effects on cardiac risk factors might promote a different biological effect *in vivo*. Both tamoxifen and raloxifene have shown some promise in reducing cardiac end-points in randomized trials to evaluate non-cardiac end-points (breast cancer and postmenopausal bone loss, respectively). Formal evaluation of raloxifene in coronary prevention is currently underway.

Table 4.1
Summary of the randomized evidence regarding the use of HRT in coronary artery disease

Study	HRT	Route	Primary/ secondary	Relative risk of AMI	Sample size
HERS Hulley *et al* 1998	CEE /MPA	Oral	Secondary	0.99	2769
WHI Roussow *et al* 2002	CEE/MPA	Oral	Primary	1.29	16608
WHI Anderson *et al* 2004	CEE	Oral	Primary	0.91	10739
PHASE Clarke *et al* 2002	17-β-oestradiol	Transdermal	Secondary	1.29	255
WEST Viscoli *et al* 2001	17-β-oestradiol	Oral	Pre-symptomatic	0.8	664
ESPRIT Cherry *et al* 2002	Oestradiol valerate	Oral	Secondary	0.99	1017

AMI, acute myocardial infarction; CEE, conjugated equine oestrogen; MPA, Medroxyprogesterone acetate; Presymptomatic, prior history of atherosclerotic disease

The risk of myocardial infarction was increased by first generation oral contraceptives, however, with the lower oestrogen doses used today the risk is extremely small unless the patient is older than 35 and/or smokes. Newer progestogens, such as gestodene, desogestrel, and norgestimate, have beneficial effects on lipoprotein levels but may increase thromboembolic complications. Data regarding the effect on heart disease risk are conflicting.

To summarize, once coronary disease has developed, the use of HRT is effectively usually contraindicated. Whether HRT used at the time of menopause might reduce subsequent risk remains possible and biologically plausible. It is, however, unlikely that this hypothesis will ever be appropriately tested. Whatever the effect, negative or positive, the size is likely to be negligible because of the low incidence of events in this population and HRT can be used safely on low-to-average risk women for symptom control.

The evaluation of chest pain in women

It is a widely held belief that cardiac symptoms in women are less 'typical' than in men; although in some studies women appear more likely to have nausea and jaw, back or neck pain, or palpitations and are less likely to report diaphoresis than men. Other work has, however, suggested that when compared to coronary angiography, women and men suffer typical and atypical symptoms to the same extent. In women presenting with a myocardial infarction, symptoms other than chest pain often predominate and this can lead to delay in receiving prompt treatment. Women are more likely to experience:

- neck and shoulder pain
- abdominal pain
- nausea
- vomiting
- fatigue and dyspnoea.

Once chest pain has developed women take longer to reach hospital, partly because of a longer time delay in calling for help (the reasons for which are obscure), and also because attending healthcare staff are less likely to attribute symptoms to an acute infarction.

Diagnostic tests in women

The resting ECG reveals a higher prevalence of repolarization (ST–T waves) abnormalities in women, thereby making ECG diagnosis more challenging. Exercise treadmill testing has a higher false positive rate in women than in men and a greater proportion of women fail to achieve a diagnostic workload. The addition of echocardiography to electrocardiography stress testing markedly improves accuracy. A meta-analysis has shown that isotope scintigraphy (with exercise testing) has 78% sensitivity and 64% specificity in diagnosis of coronary disease in women. Recent advances, especially gated wall motion analysis, mean much of the former inaccuracy of this technique can be overcome. Women are more likely than men to experience vascular and renal complications from diagnostic angiography, possibly due to advanced age, higher prevalence of diabetes, and smaller body size but the incidence of myocardial infarction, stroke and death are similar.

Treatment of myocardial infarction

Gender differences are observed following acute myocardial infarction with women experiencing a different clinical presentation and hospital course after acute coronary syndromes. In particular there may be gender differences in the response to both medical and procedural therapies. Most studies have reported near equal rates of angioplasty and bypass surgery among catheterized patients suggesting that differences in access to treatment disappear once disease is documented angiographically.

Following a myocardial infarction women tend to suffer more early complications and high-risk markers, such as tachycardia, basal crepitations and heart block. Despite this women are less likely to receive thrombolysis, and when it is administered, they receive it later than men. The post-thrombolysis complication rates, particularly recurrent myocardial infarction and haemorrhagic strokes, are higher in women. Some studies have shown that men may benefit more than women when treated with acetyl cholinesterase inhibitors in this setting, but beta-blockers clearly showed a substantial improvement in post infarction survival in both genders. Coronary revascularization is indicated in acute ST elevation myocardial infarction either as the primary mode of restoring blood flow as an alternative to thrombolysis or for ongoing ischaemia following thrombolysis. There is general acceptance that, where possible, primary infarct angioplasty is the preferred mode of reperfusion and this is particularly true for women. Gender-specific analysis of the PAMI study suggests that complications and mortality among women are considerably lower when using a percutaneous coronary intervention (PCI) than with thrombolysis, partly due to a lower risk of intracranial haemorrhage. In contrast, following a myocardial infarction not characterized by ST elevation, an aggressive strategy of revascularization does not seem to benefit women (but it does benefit men). Further examination suggests the reason is the very low number of surgical revascularizations performed in women compared to men. Virtually all PCI studies note a greater prevalence of co-morbidities in women, including:

- advanced age
- hypertension
- congestive heart failure
- diabetes
- severe noncardiac disease
- hypercholesterolemia.

The proportional risk of death from procedural complications is greater in women. Gender differences in outcome from bypass surgery are well established and are similar to PCI. The mortality of women is higher by a factor of about 40%. This is explained by differences in co-morbidity, age and body habitus. Women have a lower likelihood of being free of angina than men and experience greater physical disability and less return to work.

Gender bias

There is no doubt that women are less likely to receive investigation and timely treatment than men with a similar presenting syndrome. What remains unclear is whether this represents institutional sexism among the medical establishment or if it is a result of the different demographic features observed in women, in particular their older age and the high prevalence of co-morbid diseases, such as diabetes and hypertension. Men with a positive exercise test are 6.3 times more likely to be referred for coronary angiography than women, leading to concern that females are receiving sub-optimal care. The increased awareness of cardiovascular disease in women may ultimately improve the situation.

Conclusion

Acute myocardial infarction is one of the most common causes of death in women in the western world. Any attempt to reduce long-term disease burden needs to address the needs of the female population. The aggressive treatment of cardiac risk factors remains the cornerstone of cardiac protection and, in this respect, focussing on a case-finding approach to risk-factor control and public education are vital. Smoking is a particular concern in young women and urgently needs to be addressed. The use of female sex hormones has not realized the hopes that this would form part of a cardioprotective strategy in women and indeed in those with established disease these agents are now considered contraindicated. Although the diagnostic and therapeutic strategies of CAD are based on principles common to both sexes, differences exist in risk factors, clinical presentation, hormonal influences, diagnostic evaluation, treatment and outcomes of interventions for coronary artery diseases. Women have more difficulty accessing cardiac care and increased education of prospective patients and healthcare professionals is essential to redress this inequity.

Further reading

American Heart Association. *Heart disease and stroke statistics – 2003 update.* Dallas, TX: American Heart Association, 2002. http://www.americanheart.org

Anderson GL, Limacher M, Assaf AR *et al.* Effects of conjugated equine estrogen in postmenopausal women with hysterectomy: the Women's Health Initiative randomized controlled trial. *JAMA* 2004; **291**: 1701–12.

British Heart Foundation: *Heart disease and stroke statistics – 2004 update.* London: British Heart Foundation, 2004. http://www.bhf.org.uk

Cherry N, Gilmour K, Hannaford P *et al.* Oestrogen therapy for prevention of reinfarction in postmenopausal women: a randomised placebo controlled trial. *Lancet.* 2002; **360**: 2001–8.

Clarke SC, Kelleher J, Lloyd-Jones H *et al.* A study of hormone replacement therapy in postmenopausal women with ischaemic heart disease: the Papworth HRT atherosclerosis study. *Br J Obstet Gynaecol* 2002; **109**: 1056–62.

Edwards FH, Carey JS, Grover FL *et al.* Impact of gender on coronary bypass operative mortality. *Ann Thorac Surg* 1998; **66**: 125–31.

Espeland M, Marcovina S, Miller V *et al.* Effects of postmenopausal hormonal replacement in lipoprotein (a) concentrations. *Circulation* 1998; **97**: 979–86.

Grundy SM, Pasternak R, Greenland P *et al.* Assessment of cardiovascular risk by use of multiple risk-factor assessment equations: A statement for healthcare professionals from the American Heart Association and American College of Cardiology. *Circulation* 1999; **100**: 1481–92.

Hamelin BA, Methot J, Arsenault M. Influence of the menstrual cycle on the timing of acute coronary events in premenopausal women. *Am J Med* 2003, **114**. 599–602.

Hayes SN, Taler SJ. Hypertension in women: Current understanding of gender differences. *Mayo Clin Proc* 1998; **73**: 157–65.

Hulley S, Grady D, Bush T *et al*: Randomised trial of oestrogen plus progestin for secondary prevention of coronary heart disease in postmenopausal women. *JAMA* 1998; **280**: 605.

Kaplan JR, Manuck SB, Anthony MS. Premenopausal social status and hormone exposure predict postmenopausal atherosclerosis in female monkeys. *Obstet Gynecol* 2002; **99**: 381–8.

Knopp RH. Risk factors for coronary artery disease in women. *Am J Cardiol* 2002; **89**: 28E–34E.

Kwok Y, Kic C, Grady D *et al*: Meta-analysis of exercise testing to detect coronary artery disease in women. *Am J Cardiol* 1999; **83**: 660–6.

Lawlor D, Ebrahim S, Davey Smith G. Role of endogenous oestrogen in aetiology of coronary heart disease: analysis of age related trends in coronary heart disease and breast cancer in England and Wales and Japan. *BMJ* 2002; **325**: 311–12.

Lerner DJ, Kannel WB. Patterns of coronary heart disease morbidity and mortality in the sexes: 26-year follow-up of the Framingham population. *Am Heart J* 1986; **111**: 383–90.

Lloyd GW, Patel NR, McGing E *et al.* Does angina vary with the menstrual cycle in women with premenopausal coronary artery disease? *Heart* 2000; **84**: 189–92.

Malenka DJ, O' Rourke D, Miller MA *et al.* Cause of in-hospital death in 12,232 consecutive patients undergoing percutaneous transluminal coronary angioplasty. *Am Heart J* 1999; **137**: 632–8.

Manson JE, Hu FB, Rich-Edwards JW *et al.* A prospective study of walking as compared with vigorous exercise in the prevention of coronary heart disease in women. *N Engl J Med* 1999; **341**: 650–8.

Milani RV, Lavie CJ, Cassidy MM. Effects of cardiac rehabilitation and exercise training programs on depression in patients after major coronary events. *Am Heart J* 1996; **132**: 726–32.

Mosca L, Manson JE, Sutherland SE *et al.* Cardiovascular disease in women: A statement for healthcare professionals from AHA. *Circulation* 1997; **96**: 2468–82.

Ridker PM, Hennekens CH, Buring JE, Rifai NC. C-reactive protein and other markers of inflammation in the prediction of cardiovascular disease in women. *N Engl J Med* 2000; **342**: 836–43.

Rossouw JE, Anderson GL, Prentice RL. Risks and benefits of estrogen plus progestin in healthy postmenopausal women: principal results From the Women's Health Initiative randomized controlled trial. *JAMA* 2002; **288**: 321–33.

Sacks F, Tonkin A, Shepherd J *et al.* Effect of Pravastatin on Coronary Disease Events in Subgroups Defined by Coronary Risk Factors. *Circulation* 2000; **102**: 1893–900.

Tunstall-Pedoe H, Morrison C, Woodward M *et al.* Sex differences in myocardial infarction and coronary deaths in the Scottish MONICA population of Glasgow 1985-1991: Presentation, diagnosis, treatment, and 28 day care fatality of 3,991 events in men and 1551 events in women. *Circulation* 1996; **93**: 1981–92.

Viscoli CM, Brass LM, Kernan WN *et al.* A clinical trial of estrogen-replacement therapy after ischemic stroke. *N Engl J Med* 2001; **345**: 1243–9.

5 Stroke

Catrina Bain and Matthew Walters

Introduction

Stroke occurs when circulation of blood in the brain is disturbed, leading to focal (or at times global) loss of cerebral function. In the majority (80%) of cases, this disturbance arises as a consequence of arterial occlusion. Less commonly the clinical syndrome may occur as a result of haemorrhage from a cerebral vessel into the surrounding brain tissue. If the resulting neurological deficit resolves fully within 24 hours, the event is termed a 'transient ischaemic attack' (TIA).

Stroke is among the most important causes of severe disability in the Western world, and is the third leading cause of death (after coronary heart disease and cancer) in most Western countries. The condition has a profound social and economic effect on the affected patient, their relatives and society as a whole. In the UK, for example, stroke directly consumes a substantial proportion of health service resources, and is responsible for many less obvious costs (such as loss of income and long-term residential and non-residential care – see Chapters 9 and 10). Although stroke patients account for only 2% of hospital discharges in the UK, 4.6% of all UK health service costs are used in their care and they account for 7% of UK hospital bed-days. Whereas the considerable financial costs to the health service are relatively easy to measure, the enormous burden borne by society as a whole is more difficult to estimate. Approximately one-quarter of stroke patients are below retirement age, leading to direct loss of income and to indirect costs, such as reduced national productivity. In addition, much of the long-term care afforded to patients disabled by stroke is provided by family members, and to date little effort has been made to define the level and specific nature of the burden upon relatives of stroke patients.

The burden of stroke

A strong relationship exists between stroke incidence and increasing age. Rates of stroke increase in a consistent manner in each decade of life after the sixth (Figure 5.1). Although stroke is a leading cause of death and long-term disability in women, incidence of stroke is lower in premenopausal women than in age-matched men. After the menopause, however, risk of stroke increases in women until the gender discrepancy eventually disappears. Whereas incidence and prevalence of stroke are similar in both sexes women are more likely to die of stroke, with women accounting for approximately 60% of all stroke deaths. One in five 50-year-old Caucasian women in the Western world will develop stroke during their lifetime. Despite the huge burden of cerebrovascular disease among the female population, historically stroke has attracted comparatively little research funding compared with other major illnesses, such as heart disease and cancer. Fortunately this deficit has been partially addressed in recent years, as the relationship between menopause and incidence of stroke has generated interest in the role of female sex hormones in protection from cerebrovascular disease.

The challenge of reducing the burden of stroke on society is huge, and will not be met solely by improving the initial and secondary preventive care offered to patients with stroke. Primary stroke prevention is potentially the most effective method of reducing overall stroke-related morbidity and

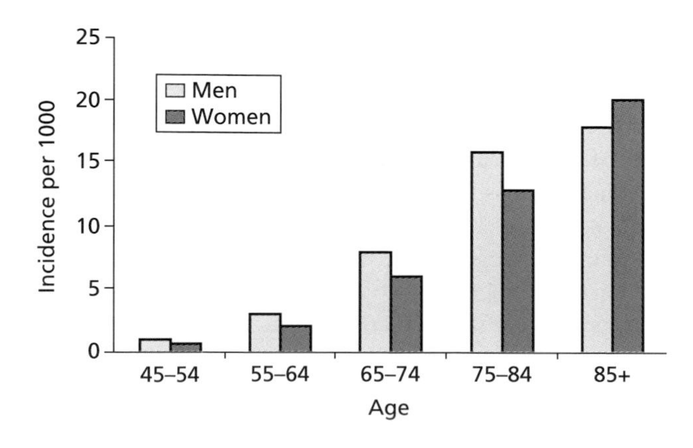

Figure 5.1 Incidence of stroke (per 1000 per year) with age by gender

mortality, and the importance of risk factor intervention, such as blood pressure control, smoking cessation and appropriate management of predisposing cardiac disease, has become apparent over recent years. Advances in our knowledge of the relationship between menopause, hormone replacement therapy (HRT) and stroke will also play a part in reducing the impact of this common and devastating condition. Although both primary and secondary preventive strategies have improved, the progressive rise in the number of elderly people in Western countries leads to the conclusion that the burden of stroke will remain a significant health and socioeconomic problem for many years to come.

Symptoms

Patients with stroke typically experience symptoms characterized by sudden onset of a neurological deficit. The more common presentations include loss of motor power or sensation involving the face, arm and leg on one side of the body. Patients may experience loss of ability to speak, comprehend speech, read or write due to involvement of the areas of brain responsible for the processing of language. Disturbances of blood flow through the brainstem and cerebellum may cause vertigo, ataxia, dysarthria, dysphagia and palsies of lower cranial nerves. Large strokes in this area cause extensive neurological deficits, including reduction in level of consciousness and quadriparesis. The clinical spectrum of stroke is wide and varied, and the initial diagnosis may prove challenging. Modern management of cerebrovascular disease makes use of a variety of imaging modalities that enable clinicians to identify the nature and aetiology of the patient's symptoms, and so elicit optimal treatment.

Investigation

The diagnosis of stroke usually begins with identification of a focal neurological deficit. The initial encounter with the patient should achieve several aims:

- confirmation of the vascular nature of the lesion
- identification of the location and extent of the cerebral damage
- institution of appropriate treatment to minimize ongoing cerebral damage
- an indication of the likely aetiology of the event.

Subsequent interaction with the patient should involve:

- institution of appropriate secondary preventive measures to avert subsequent vascular events
- recognition of existing co-morbidities and anticipation of development of known complications of stroke disease, such as deep venous thrombosis.

Considerations in the diagnosis of stroke

The main differential diagnoses of cerebrovascular disease are seizure activity and migraine. In the elderly, systemic infections, such as urinary tract sepsis, may present with neurological symptoms that may be confused with cerebral ischaemia. Sufficient information to exclude these possibilities can usually be obtained from a detailed history from the patient or witnesses. Further alternative causes of focal neurological deficit include cerebral space-occupying lesions, such as subdural haemorrhage or tumour; metabolic disturbances, such as hypo- or hyperglycaemia; infections, such as encephalitis; or cerebral abscess, hypertensive encephalopathy, syncope or demyelination. In many cases, further clarification with brain imaging or blood tests may be required before the vascular nature of the symptoms can be identified.

Having identified cerebrovascular disease as the likely underlying pathology, attention should be turned to the nature of the vascular lesion. It is important to distinguish cerebral haemorrhage from cerebral infarction at an early stage, due to profound differences in the management of these conditions. Many scales designed to allow differentiation of ischaemic stroke from cerebral haemorrhage on clinical grounds have been proposed; however none has been shown to be reliable, and in some cases they may be misleading. Brain imaging is necessary so that cerebral haemorrhage can be reliably excluded. Conventional X-ray computed tomography (CT) will reliably detect intracerebral haemorrhage within two weeks of stroke (Figures 5.2 and 5.3). However, if more than two weeks has elapsed since ictus, involutional change within the intracerebral haematoma makes haemorrhage hard to distinguish from infarct using CT scanning, and magnetic resonance imaging (MRI) may be required.

In most cases, clinical examination allows reasonable estimation of the location and extent of cerebral damage following stroke. The majority of symptoms arising as a result of stroke can be attributed to dysfunction of an identifiable area of brain, for example monoparesis following infarction of a discrete area of motor cortex. Other symptoms arising as a result of stroke may be less easy to categorize: isolated dysarthria, vertigo, confusion and cognitive disturbance (such as amnesia) may all reflect focal neurological dysfunction but may also occur as a result of a more diffuse cerebral insult.

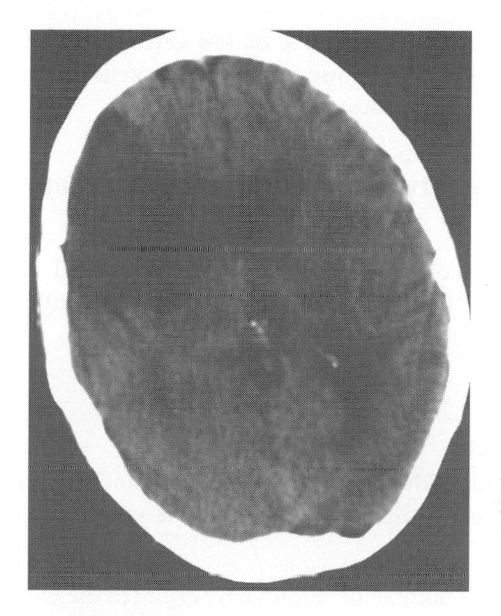

Figure 5.2 Computed tomography scan of cerebral infarction

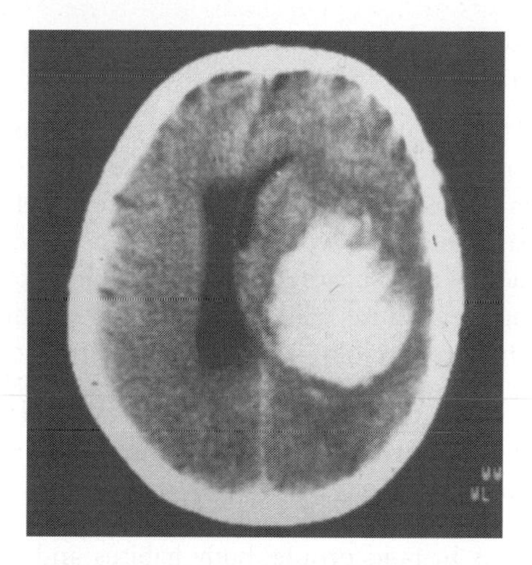

Figure 5.3 Computed tomography scan of cerebral haemorrhage

Localization of cerebral infarction may yield information concerning the underlying aetiology of the stroke, which in turn may influence further management. Patients with ischaemic stroke in the carotid territory and ipsilateral severe carotid artery stenosis should be considered for carotid endarterectomy. Patients with infarction in areas of brain susceptible to reduced perfusion (in the context of low cerebral blood flow) should be investigated for underlying causes of severe hypotension, such as paroxysmal dysrhythmias or silent myocardial infarction.

Relationships between menopause, vascular risk factors and stroke

Stroke is uncommon in premenopausal women, and its incidence rises sharply following the menopause. In addition to age, other significant risk factors for stroke in women are:

- hypertension
- diabetes
- cigarette smoking
- a constellation of atherogenic metabolic and biochemical abnormalities seen in postmenopausal women, termed the 'menopause metabolic syndrome'.

Over recent years a number of studies have explored the mechanisms through which menopause may influence blood pressure and biochemistry to increase stroke risk.

Menopause and hypertension

Hypertension is the single most important risk factor for stroke. The relationship between blood pressure and stroke risk is strong, with an exponential rise in risk as pressure increases. Systolic blood pressure is higher in young (<40 years) men than women, but this relationship reverses by the age of 60. Longitudinal data suggest an increase in blood pressure within the first year following menopause, achieving statistical significance within five years. Intervention to reduce blood pressure in postmenopausal women as well as in men is the most effective primary prevention strategy known, reducing stroke risk by approximately 40%.

Menopause and the atherogenic state

A variety of changes in lipid profile, body habitus and rheological factors occur following menopause, all of which may contribute to the development of vascular disease. Weight gain, increased plasma low-density lipoprotein concentration and changes in coagulation factors are well-recognized contributors to an atherogenic state, and all occur in postmenopausal women. With regard to the cerebral circulation, these alterations may contribute to the increased thickness of the wall of the carotid arteries in postmenopausal compared with premenopausal women. They may also be involved in the reduced reactivity of cerebral resistance vessels, such as the carotid and middle cerebral arteries, as reported in cross-sectional studies of pre- and postmenopausal women.

Effects of HRT on the brain

Effect of oestrogen on cerebral ischaemia

In experimental models of stroke, oestrogen exerts a neuroprotective effect, attenuating the severity of brain injury caused by experimental occlusion of the rat middle cerebral artery. This effect is apparent at both low (physiological) oestrogen levels and following administration of supra-physiological doses. The mechanism behind this observation is not clear; receptor-mediated transcription of genes that may prevent ischaemic cell death has been proposed. However, interaction with neuronal growth factors or oestrogen-mediated improvement in vascular endothelial function are also plausible hypotheses.

Effect of HRT on blood pressure and cerebral blood vessels

A number of studies have demonstrated the effects of postmenopausal oestrogen deficiency and HRT on the cerebral vasculature. In the post-menopausal state, cerebral vascular resistance increases with consequent modest reduction in cerebral perfusion. Following oestrogen administration this increased resistance is reduced, with consequent increase in cerebral blood flow.

Prospective studies of HRT in vascular health and disease

Effect of HRT on stroke risk in healthy women

The Women's Health Initiative (WHI) Study of 16 608 healthy post-menopausal women with an intact uterus compared continuous combined HRT (medroxyprogesterone acetate and conjugated equine oestrogen) with placebo over a long follow-up period. An elevated risk of stroke was seen in the recipients of active treatment, 29 per 10 000 person years *vs* 21 per 10 000 person years in the placebo group (Figure 5.4). These findings were reproduced in a smaller study of 10 739 hysterectomized women randomized to receive oestrogen alone or placebo, followed up over almost seven years. In this trial HRT was also associated with an approximately 40% increase in risk of stroke, not influenced by age or demographic characteristics.

Women with cerebrovascular disease

Similar trials have been conducted in women with a history of vascular disease. The Women's Estrogen and Stroke Trial (WEST) was a secondary

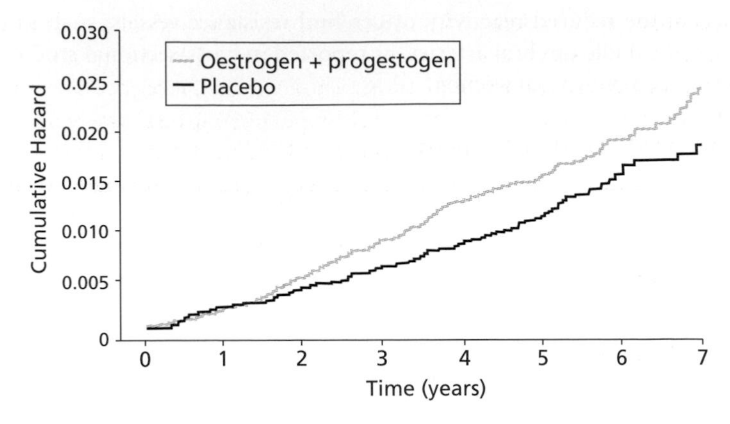

Figure 5.4 Stroke incidence in the WHI study of continuous combined HRT. Reproduced with permission

prevention study of 664 women randomized to either oestrogen or placebo early after ischaemic stroke or TIA. A trend towards increased risk of fatal stroke and poorer function outcome following non-fatal stroke was seen in the recipients of active treatment.

Women with coronary arterial disease

The Heart Estrogen Replacement Study (HERS) investigated the effect of continuous combined HRT in women with established coronary arterial disease. Although primarily intended to study coronary events, data on stroke incidence during follow-up were also analyzed. As expected the incidence of stroke was higher in this population than in healthy women. There were 12 events per 1000 patient years in the placebo group and 15 events per 1000 patient years in the treated group. Although the risk of stroke did not differ between the two groups over the full duration of follow-up, a modest increase in risk of stroke conferred by active treatment was reported within the first year of randomization.

Conclusion

Risk of stroke increases sharply after menopause, and the burden of stroke in the postmenopausal population is huge. Despite data from preclinical studies suggesting a neuroprotective effect of oestrogen, as well as a number of mechanistic studies in postmenopausal women that suggest a beneficial effect of oestrogen administration on cerebral vascular function, data from large randomized controlled trials suggest a negative impact of HRT on the overall risk of stroke. It is unlikely that the observed increased stroke risk is attributable to a deleterious effect of HRT upon the cerebral vasculature, and the mechanism that underlies the increase in stroke is undefined. Similarly, whether this increased risk of stroke may be modified by the type of HRT provided, the dose or the route of administration has not been well studied. Until these questions are addressed, healthy postmenopausal women taking HRT should be considered at slightly increased risk of stroke and this should be borne in mind when decisions to initiate such treatment are made. Women with a prior history of stroke or TIA should be counselled regarding the increased risk to which they would be exposed by HRT, and should a stroke or TIA occur in a woman taking HRT, treatment withdrawal is advised.

Further reading

Anderson GL, Limacher M. Effects of conjugated equine estrogen in postmenopausal women with hysterectomy: The Women's Health Initiative Randomized Controlled Trial. *JAMA* 2004; **29**: 1701–12.

Bousser MG. Stroke in women: the 1997 Paul Dudley White International Lecture. *Circulation* 1999; **99**: 463–7.

Celani MG, Righetti E, Migliacci R *et al.* Comparability and validity of two clinical scores in the early differential diagnosis of acute stroke. *BMJ* 1994; **308**: 1674–6.

Collins R, Peto R, MacMahon S *et al.* Blood pressure, stroke and coronary heart disease. Part 2, short-term reductions in blood pressure: overview of randomised drug trials in their epidemiological context. *Lancet* 1990; **335**: 827–38.

Dobs AS, Nieto FJ, Szklo M *et al.* Risk factors for popliteal and carotid wall thicknesses in the atherosclerosis risk in communities (ARIC) study. *Am J Epidemiol* 1999; **150**: 1055–67.

Gangar KF, Vyas S, Whitehead M *et al.* Pulsatility index in internal carotid artery in relation to transdermal oestradiol and time since menopause. *Lancet* 1991; **338**: 839–42.

Goldstein LBM, Adams RM, Becker KM *et al.* Primary prevention of ischemic stroke: a statement for healthcare professionals from the Stroke Council of the American Heart Association. *Circulation* 2001; **103**: 163–82.

Hulley S, Grady D, Bush T *et al.* Randomized trial of estrogen plus progestin for secondary prevention of coronary heart disease in postmenopausal women. Heart and Estrogen/progestin Replacement Study (HERS) Research Group. *JAMA* 1998; **280**: 605–13.

Hurn PD, Macrae IM. Estrogen as a neuroprotectant in stroke. *J Cerebral Blood Flow Metab* 2000; **20**: 631–52.

Isard PA, Forbes JF. The cost of stroke to the national health service in Scotland. *Cerebrovascular Diseases* 1992; **2**: 47–50.

Kastrup A, Dichgans J, Niemeier M, Schabet M. Changes of cerebrovascular CO_2 reactivity during normal aging. *Stroke* 1998; **29**: 1311–14.

Landahl S, Bengtsson C, Sigurdsson JA. Age-related changes in blood pressure. *Hypertension* 1986; **11**: 1044–9.

Martin J, Meltzer H, Elliott D. *The prevalence of disability among adults.* London: HMSO, 1988.

Murray CJ, Lopez AD. Mortality by cause for eight regions of the world: Global Burden of Disease Study. *Lancet* 1997; **349**: 1269–76.

Penotti M, Nencioni T, Gabrielli L *et al.* Blood flow variations in internal carotid and middle cerebral arteries induced by postmenopausal hormone replacement therapy. *Am J Obstet Gynecol* 1993; **169**: 1226–32.

Reimer W. The burden of caregiving in partners of long-term stroke survivors. *Stroke* 1998; **29**: 1605–11.

Spencer CP, Godsland IF, Stevenson JC. Is there a menopausal metabolic syndrome? *Gynecol Endocrinol* 1997; **11**: 341–55.

Viscoli CM, Brass LM, Kernan WN *et al.* A clinical trial of estrogen-replacement therapy after ischemic stroke. *New Engl J Med* 2001; **345**: 1243–9.

Weir CJ, Murray GD, Adams FG *et al.* Poor accuracy of stroke scoring systems for differential clinical diagnosis of intracranial haemorrhage and infarction. *Lancet* 1994; **344**: 999–1002.

Writing Group for the Women's Health Initiative Investigators. Risks and benefits of estrogen plus progestin in healthy postmenopausal women: principal results from the women's health initiative randomized controlled trial. *JAMA* 2002; **288**: 321–33.

6 Osteoporosis

William D Fraser

Introduction

Osteoporosis is a systemic disease that results in an increased risk of fractures due to a reduction in bone mass and quality. Based on bone mineral density (BMD) measurement (Table 6.1), the World Health Organization definitions, applied to postmenopausal women, results in 30% of this population being classified as having osteoporosis. Severe osteoporosis is defined as the

Table 6.1
World Health Organization definitions

Normal
Where an individual has a BMD value between −1SD and +1SD of the young adult mean (T score −1 to +1)

Osteopenia
Where an individual has a BMD reduced between −1 and −2.5SDs from the young adult mean (T score −1 to −2.5)

Osteoporosis
Where an individual has a BMD reduced by equal to or more than −2.5SDs from the young adult mean (T score −2.5 or lower)

presence of a fragility or minimal trauma fracture (fracture after a fall from a chair or standing) and low BMD (T score<–2.5). Although BMD is a major contributor to risk, other factors including age, body mass index (BMI), falls, bone quality and the rates of bone resorption and formation play a part in determining whether a patient will suffer a fracture.

Extent of the problem

The prevalence of osteoporosis has been calculated using the NHANES database and there is a clear association with increasing age. Hip BMD classifies 20% of 65–69 year olds as having osteoporosis, increasing to just over 50% in those aged >79 years. Fracture incidence increases with age, with the greatest increase in hip, followed by vertebral then wrist fracture. A two-fold increase in fracture risk is observed for each one standard deviation reduction in BMD of hip and spine. Hip fractures are more common in Caucasians than other ethnic groups and variation in fracture rates may reflect racial/genetic differences. Fifty percent of postmenopausal women will experience an osteoporosis-related fracture during their lifetime. Population demographics predict that the number of osteoporotic fractures will double by 2040.

Pathology and effects of ageing and lack of oestrogen

Sex steroids are major contributors to the production and maintenance of skeletal health. Oestrogen is required during bone formation and the achievement of peak bone mass. Falling oestrogen production at the menopause is associated with a significant increase in bone remodelling with resorption predominating over formation. Remodelling rates double at the menopause, triple 13 years later and remain elevated thereafter in women with osteoporosis. This imbalance in bone metabolism results in loss of bone from the menopause into later life. Both cortical and trabecular bone are lost. There is increased intra-cortical porosity and decreased cortical thickness. Trabecular thinning, perforation and loss of connectivity occur.

Fracture risk increases with age independent of BMD, with the risk of hip fracture being two-fold greater at 75 years than 65 years in the presence of a hip BMD T score of –2.5. The continuing high bone-remodelling rate in women with osteoporosis is a major factor underlying this increased risk.

The relative importance of peak bone mass and subsequent rate of bone loss is still being defined but it is clear that premature menopause and prolongation of the period of altered bone remodelling results in earlier onset of osteoporosis and fracture.

A significant increase in plasma ionized calcium, decrease in gastro-intestinal absorption and renal tubular resorption of calcium without a significant change in parathyroid hormone (PTH) or vitamin D is observed from one year post-menopause. This combination is in keeping with data indicating an increase in the PTH set-point for calcium following the menopause. The postmenopausal increase in bone resorption may indicate an increased bone cell sensitivity to PTH with resultant stimulation of bone remodelling. Blunting of the endogenous circadian rhythm of PTH with a decrease in the nocturnal rise may also contribute to the overall catabolic effect of PTH on bone with ageing. Gradual loss of growth hormone secretion with age may also alter the calcium set-point and bone cell sensitivity to PTH.

Decreased sun exposure and a reduced intake of foods containing calcium and vitamin D in the elderly can result in relative vitamin D/calcium deficiency and subsequent secondary hyperparathyroidism, which will promote increased bone resorption.

Symptoms and signs

No single symptom or clinical sign can unequivocally diagnose osteoporosis. The majority of women with osteoporosis will not know they have the condition. The physical findings most likely to indicate the presence of osteoporosis or a spinal fracture are weight <51kg, tooth count <20, rib–pelvis distance <2 finger-breadths, wall–occiput distance >0cm, and self reported humped back. Exaggerated kyphosis is not always associated with osteoporosis and is more usually the result of degenerative disc disease.

A common presentation is overt fracture with pain. In women aged 50–65 years, a Colles' fracture of the wrist, usually the result of a fall on outstretched hands, is often the first sign. Sudden onset of acute severe back pain in the mid thoracic or lumbar spine with a history of mild or no trauma is a common presentation. In older women hip fractures are sustained following a fall from standing. The type of fracture – inter-trochanteric, femoral neck or sub-capital – depends on the angle and type of fall.

In Finland the number of patients admitted for treatment of low-trauma ankle fracture has increased from 369 in 1970 to 1545 in 2000 (319% increase). If this trend continues, there will be about three times more low-trauma ankle fractures in Finland in 2030 than in 2000. This increase cannot be explained simply by demographic changes and raises questions about whether increased mobility of elderly populations increases the risk of minor falls, accidents and fractures.

Impact on women's lives

Many women with low BMD may never manifest any signs of osteoporosis or experience a fracture. Knowing they have a low BMD, however, can have significant effects because of fear of future fractures and alteration of daily life to prevent falls and fractures. Negative effects of osteoporosis on quality of life (QoL) have been demonstrated even in the absence of known fractures. Lower QoL scores were noted with decreasing BMD. Height loss and kyphosis were associated with difficulty in daily activities, alteration of daily routines and fear for the future. The negative impact of osteoporosis on QoL was related more to physical manifestations than to BMD alone. Other psychological effects have been reported in women with osteoporosis, eg:

- stress
- sadness
- anger
- denial.

Increased mortality is associated with osteoporosis and for each one standard deviation that BMD is decreased, mortality risk is increased 1.5-fold. One in three women will suffer a hip fracture by 80 years and, following a hip fracture, between 25–30% of patients will die within 3–6 months. A study of 160 000 hip fractures in men and women aged over 50 years calculated that causally related deaths (directly or indirectly related to the fracture) comprised 17–32% of deaths and accounted for more than 1.5% of all deaths in this population. Excess mortality is associated with both hip and vertebral fracture but this may be secondary to other medical conditions and general health unrelated to osteoporosis. The increased mortality following hip fracture remains for 6–12 months following the fracture. Early operative intervention (within five days of fracture) may improve survival and QoL.

In older patients hip fractures have a marked effect on QoL and may result in admission to nursing homes or the requirement for additional assistance in daily living. Eighty percent of older women surveyed (>75% having experienced two or more falls, or one fall resulting in hospital admission and one hip without previous surgery) stated they would rather be dead than experience the loss of independence that could result from a hip fracture.

Who, how and when to investigate

Population screening using only bone densitometry has a low sensitivity for future fracture risk and is not merited. A case-finding strategy based on clinical criteria to identify subjects for BMD measurement and further investigation is recommended. Many guidelines exist, with similar criteria for referral for BMD measurement and the value of these has been assessed (Kayan *et al* 2003). The Royal College of Physicians (RCP) guidelines performed well in this independent assessment and can be recommended.

X-rays may detect a reduction in bone mass as an incidental finding but a

30–40% reduction in mass is required before this is obvious on a radiograph. X-rays can be helpful in detecting the presence and subsequent deterioration of a fracture; but in future the use of high-resolution fan-beam Dual X-ray Absorptiometry (DXA) could provide quantitative BMD, and visual examination of images will permit assessment of vertebral fractures.

A thorough diagnostic work-up of patients with proven osteoporosis is required. It is essential to rule out secondary causes of osteoporosis, especially serious diseases such as malignancy. This requires biochemical, haematological and radiological investigations (Table 6.2). Further investigations may be required depending on initial results. This approach should avoid inappropriate and ineffective prescription of expensive treatments.

Determining intervention thresholds for osteoporosis is difficult and there are few published studies to help decision-making regarding intervention. The diagnostic thresholds based on BMD have several problems and it has been suggested that intervention should be based on absolute risk of fracture, ie similar to the recommendations for lipid-lowering therapy.

Table 6.2

Investigation of osteoporosis

Biochemical
- Urea and electrolytes
- Liver function tests (including total alkaline phosphatase)
- Serum calcium, phosphate, total protein, albumin, globulin
- Thyroid function tests
- Serum and urine protein electrophoresis (may depend on globulin and ESR estimation)
- Urine calcium excretion

Haematological
- Full blood count
- Erythrocyte sedimentation rate (ESR)

Radiological
- Lateral X-rays of thoracic and lumbar spine

Therapy

Non-drug therapy

The nature of osteoporosis lends itself to a public health approach to primary prevention. Alteration of environmental factors, diet, exercise, reduction of excessive alcohol consumption and cessation of smoking could all contribute to an improvement in BMD and reduction in fracture risk. Each factor in isolation has a small or poorly quantified effect and no population level interventions have been implemented. Provision of milk to adolescent children can have a significant effect on peak BMD but little supportive government legislation exists.

Greater attempts should be made to reduce the risk of falling. Over 90% of hip fractures are associated with a fall. If falls can be avoided an individual should not suffer a fracture. Falls risk can be estimated using simple screening tests assessing visual acuity, heel–toe walking, the ability to rise from sitting, or standing up five times. Home assessment will detect dangers in the immediate environment, such as:

- loose fitting carpets/rugs
- ill-fitting shoes and slippers
- poor lighting
- inappropriate storage of household utensils
- structural risks, such as loose banisters.

General health measures, including provision of glasses, hearing aids and avoidance of sedatives, will be helpful.

Improving vision can have an effect on reducing falls. Significant reduction in recurrent falling and fractures by expediting cataract surgery in women aged over 70 who have bilateral cataracts has been demonstrated.

External hip protectors are designed to absorb and disperse the impact of a fall towards the soft tissues and keep the force on the femur below the fracture threshold. Although several studies have examined the effectiveness of hip protectors, results are conflicting and larger studies employing individual randomization have concluded that they are ineffective. In general acceptance of hip protectors is poor and fractures often occur in the group randomized to intervention when they are not using the protector. Structured education of carers, encouragement, reinforcement of benefits and the provision of several pairs of protectors can result in significant fracture reduction.

Drug therapy

Data on prevention of fractures in postmenopausal women mainly centres on the use of hormone replacement therapy (HRT). Observational studies indicate an association between HRT use and fracture reduction, and meta-analyses have concluded HRT reduces fractures. A prospective study of postmenopausal women concluded that HRT use immediately after the menopause is associated with a substantial reduction in all fractures. This study also concluded that HRT was most cost-effective in high-risk populations. This was in agreement with a study that concluded HRT, given on the basis of screening an asymptomatic population, was less cost-effective than targeting higher risk groups.

The use of HRT for prevention of chronic diseases has recently been questioned. The Women's Health Initiative (WHI) study and the Million Women Study have both provided data regarding the risks associated with long-term use of HRT. A significant increase in breast cancer risk was reported in both studies and the Million Women Study suggested that continuous combined HRT (containing oestrogen and progestogen) was associated with the highest incidence of breast cancer. Cardiovascular-associated mortality, cerebrovascular accidents and thromboembolic events were increased in the WHI study, but most women in the study were aged over 60 years (which inherently increases their risk of vascular disease).

Reducing fractures

Vertebral

In one meta-analysis, Vitamin D (combined with calcium), calcitonin, raloxifene and the bisphosphonates (etidronate, risedronate and alendronate) were all shown to significantly reduce vertebral fractures (Table 6.3). HRT in the meta-analysis did not have a significant effect on vertebral fractures because the analysis excluded the recent WHI study and the pooled estimate from randomized trials had a wide confidence interval.

Although raloxifene (60 mg daily for 24–36 months) produces only a modest increase in femoral neck and lumbar spine BMD, a significant reduction in vertebral (38–52%) but not hip fracture is observed when compared to controls (calcium and vitamin D). An additional beneficial effect of raloxifene is a 76% reduction in breast cancer incidence (mainly oestrogen receptor positive). Side-effects are mainly limited to muscle cramps and increased flushing but a more serious effect is the modest increase in the venous thrombosis risk, which is similar to the risk observed with HRT.

Strontium ranelate has been licensed as a treatment for osteoporosis. This molecule has a modest effect on biochemical markers of bone metabolism, increasing formation and decreasing resorption. The effect on BMD has to be interpreted with care as the molecular mass of strontium results in an 'artificial' increase in BMD. However both prevention and fracture studies have demonstrated a significant effect on vertebral and selected non-vertebral fracture incidence.

Recombinant human PTH (1–34) (teriparatide) has received approval for use in the USA and Europe. Injecting PTH (1–34) 20μg daily subcutaneously for 18 months significantly increased mean lumbar spine (8.6%) and femoral neck (2.1%) BMD. New vertebral fractures decreased by 65% but there was no significant decrease in hip fracture. This treatment is anabolic resulting in

Table 6.3
Drug treatments for the prevention and treatment of osteoporosis

	Spine	Hip
Bisphosphonates		
Etidronate	A	B
Alendronate	A	A
Risedronate	A	A
Calcium and Vitamin D	ND	A
Calcium	A	B
Calcitriol	A	ND
Calcitonin	A	B
Oestrogen	A	A
Selective Oestrogen Receptor Modulators (SERMS)	A	ND
Strontium ranelate	A	A
Teriparatide (parathyroid hormone)	A	ND
Vitamin D alone	A	A

(ND= not demonstrated)
The levels of evidence for the various agents detailed below are:
A = meta-analysis of RCTs or from at least one RCT/from at least one well designed controlled study without randomisation
B = from at least one other type of well designed quasi-experimental study or from well designed non-experimental descriptive studies, eg comparative studies, correlation studies, case-control studies

a significant increase in bone formation, and within one month a significant increase in the serum concentration of amino terminal pro-peptide of type 1 collagen (P1NP) is observed. PTH (1–34) is expensive costing close to £300 (US $580, Euro 430) per month and so detailed cost–benefit analysis will be required to establish its place in overall management.

Non-vertebral

Alendronate, risedronate and most recently strontium ranelate reduce non-vertebral fracture. There are minimal trial data and epidemiological evidence for other treatments and comparators, with large overlap of confidence intervals in meta-analyses.

Some treatments are more effective in certain subpopulations. The evidence for an effect of calcium plus vitamin D in patients who are vitamin D deficient, with secondary hyperparathyroidism, is much stronger than the effect in the overall elderly population. Non-vertebral fracture is significantly reduced in institutionalized patients when treated with appropriate doses of calcium (up to 1500 mg) and vitamin D (400–800 IU).

Addition of alendronate (10 mg/day) to calcium and vitamin D in a population of elderly women in long-term residential care produced a greater increase in BMD and reduction in bone turnover markers than calcium and vitamin D, without increasing side-effects. Data were not available on fracture incidence.

The WHI study reported that HRT significantly reduces hip fracture. However, several concerns regarding long-term use of HRT and the commencement of HRT in elderly women were raised by this study. In the population studied there was a predominance of adverse effects, with increased stroke, thrombosis, breast cancer and coronary heart disease over beneficial effects, such as reduction in fractures and colorectal cancer. There are no published direct comparisons of the various treatments with fracture or quality of life as outcome. Those studies that are available indicate that alendronate has a greater effect on increasing BMD or reducing bone marker production than calcitonin, risedronate and raloxifene and that little difference exists between etidronate and calcitriol.

Monitoring drug therapy

Several interventions reduce the incidence of fractures but the optimal response and duration of therapy is still unknown. Few data are available on the rate of adherence to treatment, the rate of response and the potential mechanisms to improve response to interventions. Biochemical markers of bone turnover can facilitate follow-up of patients receiving osteoporosis treatments and they can be used to detect patients who do not adhere or do not respond to treatment. Resorption markers reflect osteoclast activity and, since the majority of interventions are antiresorptive, their measurement allows prediction of reduction in fracture risk. Serum markers of resorption have reduced biological and measurement variability compared to urine markers and can follow changes with treatment with increasing accuracy. The magnitude and timing of reduction in bone markers (within weeks) is a significant advantage over the slower changes in BMD or awaiting presentation with clinical fracture as an indication of intervention efficacy. Early changes in markers of bone turnover in response to bisphosphonates predict the subsequent increase in BMD with high sensitivity, specificity and predictive values.

Conclusion

Osteoporosis is a significant public health issue. A major difficulty when analysing studies is the lack of a precise estimate of the therapeutic effect (in terms of fracture reduction) of each treatment when used in the osteoporotic population. All of the available clinical trials have different entry criteria, study populations and fracture incidence and prevalence in the controls. To obtain more standardized data would require an extremely large population database and at present this is not feasible. Further work is required to improve the value of research in this area.

Further reading

Beral V. Breast cancer and hormone-replacement therapy in the Million Women Study. *Lancet* 2003; **362**: 419–27.

Birks YF, Porthouse J, Addie C *et al.* Primary Care Hip Protector Trial Group. Randomized controlled trial of hip protectors among women living in the community. *Osteoporos Int* 2004; **15**: 701–6.

Browner WS, Seeley DG, Vogt TM, Cummings SR. Non-trauma mortality in elderly women with low bone mineral density. Study of Osteoporotic Fractures Research Group. *Lancet* 1991; **338**: 355–8.

Center JR, Nguyen TV, Schneider D *et al.* Mortality after all major types of osteoporotic fracture in men and women: an observational study. *Lancet* 1999; **353**: 878–82.

Chapurlat RD, Cummings SR. Does follow-up of osteoporotic women treated with antiresorptive therapies improve effectiveness? *Osteoporos Int* 2002; **13**: 738–44.

Chapuy MC, Pamphile R, Paris E *et al.* Combined calcium and vitamin D3 supplementation in elderly women: confirmation of reversal of secondary hyperparathyroidism and hip fracture risk: the Decalyos II study. *Osteoporos Int* 2002; **13**: 257–64.

Crandall C. Parathyroid hormone for treatment of osteoporosis. *Arch Intern Med* 2002; **162**: 2297–309.

Cranney A, Guyatt G, Griffith L *et al*; Osteoporosis Methodology Group and The Osteoporosis Research Advisory Group. Meta-analyses of therapies for post-menopausal osteoporosis. IX: Summary of meta-analyses of therapies for postmenopausal osteoporosis. *Endocr Rev* 2002; **23**: 570–8.

Cranney A, Tugwell P, Wells G, Guyatt G; The Osteoporosis Methodology Group and The Osteoporosis Research Advisory Group. Meta-analyses of therapies for postmenopausal osteoporosis. I. Systematic reviews of randomized trials in osteoporosis: introduction and methodology. *Endocr Rev* 2002; **23**: 496–507.

Deutschmann HA, Weger M, Weger W *et al.* Search for occult secondary osteoporosis: impact of identified possible risk factors on bone mineral density. *J Int Med* 2002; **252**: 389–97.

Green AD, Colon-Emeric CS, Bastian L *et al.* Does this woman have osteoporosis? *JAMA* 2004; **292**: 2890–900.

Kanis JA, Melton LJ III, Christiansen C *et al.* The diagnosis of osteoporosis. *J Bone Miner Res* 1994; **9**: 1137–41.

Kanis JA, Black D, Cooper C *et al.* A new approach to the development of assessment guidelines for osteoporosis. *Osteoporos Int* 2002; **13**: 527–36.

Kannus P, Palvanen M, Niemi S *et al.* Increasing number and incidence of low-trauma ankle fractures in elderly people: Finnish statistics during 1970–2000 and projections for the future. *Bone* 2002; **31**: 430–3.

Kayan K, de Takats D, Ashford R *et al.* Performance of clinical referral criteria for bone densitometry in patients under 65 years of age assessed by spine bone mineral density. *Postgrad Med J* 2003; **79**: 581–4.

Martin AR, Sornay-Rendu E, Chandler JM *et al.* The impact of osteoporosis on quality-of-life: the OFELY cohort. *Bone* 2002; **31**: 32–6.

Melton LJ III, Crowson CS, O'Fallon WM *et al.* Relative contributions of bone density, bone turnover, and clinical risk factors to long-term fracture prediction. *J Bone Miner Res* 2003; **18**: 312–18.

Meunier PJ, Roux C, Seeman E *et al.* The effects of strontium ranelate on the risk of vertebral fracture in women with postmenopausal osteoporosis. *N Engl J Med* 2004; **350**: 459–68.

NIH Consensus Development Panel on Osteoporosis Prevention, Diagnosis, and Therapy. Osteoporosis prevention, diagnosis, and therapy. *JAMA* 2001; **285**: 785–95.

Nordin BE, Wishart JM, Clifton PM *et al.* A longitudinal study of bone-related biochemical changes at the menopause. *Clin Endocrinol* 2004; **61**: 123–30.

Porthouse J, Cockayne S, King C *et al.* Randomised controlled trial of calcium and supplementation with cholecalciferol (vitamin D3) for prevention of fractures in primary care. *BMJ* 2005; **330**: 1003–6.

Recker R, Lappe J, Davies KM, Heaney R. Bone remodeling increases substantially in the years after menopause and remains increased in older osteoporosis patients. *J Bone Miner Res* 2004; **19**: 1628–33.

Reginster JY, Seeman E, De Vernejoul MC *et al.* Strontium ranelate reduces the risk of nonvertebral fractures in postmenopausal women with osteoporosis: TROPOS study. *J Clin Endocrinol Metab* 2005; Feb 22 [Epub ahead of print].

Rossouw JE, Anderson GL, Prentice RL *et al.* Writing Group for the Women's Health Initiative Investigators. Risks and benefits of estrogen plus progestin in healthy postmenopausal women: principal results from the Women's Health Initiative randomized controlled trial. *JAMA* 2002; **288**: 321–3.

Royal College of Physicians. *Osteoporosis: clinical guidelines for prevention and treatment. Update on pharmacological interventions and an alogorithm for management.* London: Royal College of Physicians 2000. http://www.rcplondon.ac.uk/pubs/wp_osteo_update.htm

Woolf AD, Akesson K. Preventing fractures in elderly people. *BMJ* 2003; **327**: 89–95.

7 Osteoarthritis

Sakeba N Issa and Leena Sharma

Introduction

Osteoarthritis (OA) is the most common form of arthritis and a leading cause of disability. Most disability attributable to OA comes from disease at the knee or the hip. The incidence of OA increases with age. By the age of 65, over 80% of the population have radiographic changes consistent with OA in at least one site (hands, feet, spine, knees or hips), 40% complain of arthritic symptoms and 10% report limitation in activity due to arthritis. This age-associated increase is greater in women for reasons as yet unknown.

Effects of ageing

Age is the strongest identified risk factor for the development of OA. Normal joint tissue has characteristic features, which include:

- a relatively stable cell population
- a high ratio of extracellular matrix to cells
- avascularity
- tolerance to repetitive mechanical loading in load-bearing joints.

With increasing age, chondrocytes begin to take on a yellowish colour, in part due to accumulation of lipid pigment and advanced glycation end-products. In 1999 Degroot *et al* showed that the degree of glycation is negatively correlated with the rate of proteoglycan synthesis. This suggests that advanced glycation end-products may be involved in the age-related decline of the capacity of cartilage to synthesize new tissue. Chondrocyte responsiveness to major growth factors, such as insulin-like growth factor-1 (IGF-1), also diminishes with age.

It was previously thought that OA was part of normal ageing processes; hence the historical terms 'degenerative joint disease' and 'wear-and-tear arthritis'. However normal ageing should be distinguished from OA. Changes such as subchondral bone sclerosis and focal superficial synovial inflammation are seen in OA, but not with normal ageing, whereas osteopenia and synovial atrophy are changes typical of normal ageing but not OA.

Changes seen in OA are believed to be caused by either excessive stresses on once normal joint tissues or from normal stresses acting on tissues that have been altered by systemic or local factors. OA is perpetuated by an inadequate repair response to these stresses. In the earlier stages of OA, chondrocyte proliferation and metabolic activity are increased. Matrix oedema, a consequence of repetitive mechanical stresses resulting in breakdown of the intricate collagen meshwork, is a common feature. Ultimately, the affected chondrocytes become necrotic and apoptotic.

Although chondrocyte activity is increased, it may fail to meet the demands on the joint and thus result in progressive joint damage. The diminished chondrocyte population decreases tissue capacity for sustaining the matrix proteoglycan concentration. In turn, this leads to increased tissue vulnerability to injury. Pathological changes due to OA are seen in all the articular and periarticular tissues.

It is very likely that the process leading to OA starts early in life, long before symptoms develop. Ageing may result in increased susceptibility to injury and decreased capacity for repair, further perpetuating the disease process. In addition, elements of the local joint environment, such as joint protective muscle activity, muscle strength relative to body weight, proprioception, varus-valgus laxity and meniscal condition, may become impaired and contribute to disease progression. These changes appear to be more common in women than in men. The influence of gender may be mediated through impaired joint environment and/or hormonal influences on cartilage metabolism.

Effects of hormonal factors

Gender-specific changes

The age-related increase in the prevalence of knee OA appears to be greater in women. The prevalence of radiographic findings of knee OA rises from 13% of women aged 45–49 years to 55% of women aged 80 years and older; comparable figures in men are 8% and 22%, respectively. Similar findings are found in the hand. For example, prevalence of distal interphalangeal OA involvement rises from 4% of women aged 35–39 to 73% of women aged 80 years and older (as compared to 2% and 48% in men, respectively).

In a longitudinal study, rates of incident knee OA were 1.8-fold higher in women than in men [95% confidence interval (CI) 1.0–2.7] adjusting for age, body mass index (BMI), smoking, injury, chondrocalcinosis, hand OA, and physical activity. Moreover, the gender difference in the incidence of knee, hip, and hand OA first becomes apparent during the menopause, suggesting a role of hormonal factors. Although gender appears to increase the risk of incident OA, published reports have not described a difference between men and women in the likelihood of disease progression.

Effects of oestrogen

The changes in OA incidence with age and by gender imply that oestrogen deficiency is a risk factor. Results of studies examining the relationship between oestrogen and pathogenesis of OA are conflicting. For example, in 1997 Cicuttini *et al* found that premenopausal women were less likely than postmenopausal women to have patellofemoral OA even after adjusting for potential confounders, such as age, weight, and hormone replacement therapy (adjusted OR 0.23, 95% CI 0.06–0.84). However, in 1993 Samanta *et al* found no association between oestrogen-related hormonal events, such as age at menarche or menopause and OA.

The effect of oestrogen administration has been examined in animal models and in humans. Cartilage lesions of OA were significantly less severe in the animals given oestrogen compared with those in a control group. Similarly, ovariectomized rats receiving oestrogen had a delay in the development of OA. However, studies of oestrogen replacement in women have produced conflicting results.

Overall most studies suggest that oestrogen use is associated with a lower-than-expected risk of knee and hip OA. An MRI-based study suggested that oestrogen use might prevent loss of knee articular cartilage in post-menopausal women. Also current oestrogen users have been found to be 38% less likely to have hip OA compared to non-users. There was evidence of a dose–response relationship among current oestrogen users. In current users, oestrogen for ≥10 years was associated with a greater reduction in the risk of hip OA than use for less than 10 years (OR 0.57, 95% CI 0.40–0.82 *vs* OR 0.75, 95% CI 0.46–1.24, respectively). The majority of other studies did not reach statistical significance. However, results are consistent in their direction and suggest the possibility of a protective effect of oestrogen on incident knee and hip OA.

No difference has been found between oestrogen and placebo in effect on knee pain and related disability as assessed using the Western Ontario and McMaster Universities (WOMAC) Osteoarthritis Index. The prevalence of frequent knee symptoms was similar in those assigned to receive oestrogen and placebo respectively (24.1% *vs* 26.1%; 95% CI -7.4–3.5) as were WOMAC pain scores (5.9±3.9 *vs* 6.1±3.8; 95% CI -1.2–0.8).

Symptoms and findings

The diagnosis of OA is usually clinical and is based on the age, symptoms, location and number of joints involved as well as radiographic findings. Secondary causes of OA include prior joint trauma, congenital or developmental abnormalities, other bone and joint diseases (such as rheumatoid arthritis and calcium deposition disorders), and other systemic diseases (such as diabetes mellitus and thyroid disease). More commonly OA is idiopathic. As such it may be local (confined to one joint) or generalized (commonly defined as affecting the hands and at least one major weight-bearing joint). Localized OA most commonly occurs in:

- hands (proximal and distal interphalangeal joints)
- first carpometacarpal joints
- feet (especially first metatarsophalangeal joints)
- knee
- hip
- spine (especially cervical and lumbosacral).

Symptoms include pain, stiffness, crepitus and joint swelling. Pain is the most common symptom. Pain and joint damage do not correlate as strongly as might be anticipated. This may be partly due to adaptations to chronic pain, such as activity avoidance, or may reflect the limitations of radiography to capture pain-related elements of the disease. The pain is typically worsened after activity and relieved by rest. In advanced disease, pain may come on with progressively less activity and ultimately may occur at rest. Since cartilage is not innervated, cartilage damage is not a direct cause of pain. Studies suggest that in the knee, bone pathology (eg cysts, oedema, attrition or osteophytes, which are bony outgrowths) may play a central role in pain presence and severity. Stiffness resolving within 30 minutes after a patient awakens is also a common manifestation. Often patients will complain of 'gelling' or stiffness following periods of inactivity.

Crepitus is especially common in the knee. Joint effusion, morning stiffness for longer than 30 minutes or chondrocalcinosis are characteristic of inflammatory OA. Osteophytes occurring on the distal and proximal interphalangeal joints of the hand are referred to as Heberden's and Bouchard's nodes, respectively. As the osteophytes grow, they may cause erythema of the overlying skin and significant pain. These bony growths can lead to loss of motion manifested as locking or contractures of joints, eg in the fingers and knees.

Determinants of functional impairment in knee osteoarthritis

While pain is likely to be a central factor in limiting physical function of the knee in OA, it is not the only one (Table 7.1). In the Framingham cohort, limited function was more likely to be present in conjunction with moderately severe OA and infrequent pain than with milder OA and frequent pain. Numerous cross-sectional studies and a small number of longitudinal studies have pointed to other factors, such as:

- low self-sufficiency
- obesity
- comorbidity
- depressive symptoms
- low social support
- low levels of physical activity.

We recently found that the likelihood of poor functional outcome was increased by the presence of greater varus-valgus laxity, BMI, knee pain intensity, and greater proprioceptive inaccuracy. Better mental health, self-efficiency and social support, and more aerobic exercise decreased the likelihood of poor outcome independent of pain.

Table 7.1

Factors that may influence physical function in knee OA

- Knee pain intensity
- Older age
- Greater body mass index
- Comorbid conditions
- Low physical activity
- Varus-valgus laxity
- Hip–knee–ankle malalignment
- Muscle weakness
- Proprioceptive impairment
- Depressive symptoms
- Anxiety
- Poor social support
- Low self-sufficiency

Treatment

Improving quality of life and pain relief, minimizing disability and preventing disease progression are the primary goals of treatment. No proven disease-modifying therapies exist for OA. Treatment is varied and includes both

Table 7.2
Treatment modalities for OA [Jordan 2003]

- Education
- Weight loss
- Physical therapy
  - Aerobic exercise
  - Strengthening
  - Aquatherapy
  - Ultrasound stimulation
  - Transcutaneous electrical nerve stimulation
- Occupational therapy
  - Aids
  - Orthotic devices
  - Shoe insoles
- Pharmacologic agents
  - Acetaminophen (paracetamol)
  - Nonsteriodal anti-inflammatory drugs (NSAIDs)
  - Cyclooxygenase-2 selective inhibitors (role uncertain at present)
- Topical creams
  - Capsaicin cream
  - NSAID cream
- Glucosamine chondrotin
- Tramadol
- Opioid therapy
- Intraarticular injection
  - Corticosteroids
  - Hyaluronic acid derivatives
- Surgical intervention

pharmacological and non-pharmacological modalities (Table 7.2). Management should be tailored to each patient and should take into account the individual's functional status, occupational needs, coexisting medical problems, severity of the disease and joint deformity.

Non-pharmacological interventions

The major non-pharmacological modalities used to treat OA include weight loss, aerobic exercise, exercise to maintain strength and proper footwear. Orthotics include braces, splints and insoles. The use of orthoses in the management of OA may assist in relieving pain and improving function of the affected joint. Orthoses may be used for weight-bearing joints, particularly the knee, or may be applied in hand and wrist OA. Emerging evidence suggests a potential role for urethane wedge shoe insole orthotic devices. Lateral heel wedging may decrease pain in medial compartment OA, presumably by either correcting a reducible varus deformity or by helping unload the medial compartment. Exercise may reverse some deficits in gait, flexibility and strength. Patients starting an exercise programme need to be instructed on proper footwear and taught how to gradually increase the intensity and duration of exercise so they do not cause an exacerbation of their symptoms.

A referral to physical and/or occupational therapy may be warranted in some patients. Studies have shown improvement of functional outcomes and pain scores in OA patients who have undergone a flexibility and muscle strengthening training programme. The aim of such therapy is to preserve the strength of muscle groups surrounding the diseased joints. Heat, cold, ultrasound and massage may also reduce some of the pain. Finally, psychosocial support may help to prevent physical limitations, dependency and depression.

Pharmacological interventions

In most cases non-prescription paracetamol (acetaminophen) is the first choice for pain relief in people with non-inflammatory OA. At doses up to 4 g/day, acetaminophen is generally well-tolerated. Liver toxicity may occur. However, at these doses, liver toxicity is usually seen only in patients who drink excessive amounts of alcohol.

Nonsteriodal anti-inflammatory drugs (NSAIDs) are also an appropriate management for patients with non-inflammatory and inflammatory OA. Use of over-the-counter agents, such as aspirin, ibuprofen and naproxen, and prescription agents, such as diclofenac, indomethacin and nabumetone, may be limited by adverse effects. Patients with long-term use of NSAIDs should be monitored by a physician. Among the potential toxicities of NSAIDs are:

- allergic reactions
- gastrointestinal bleeding with or without abdominal pain
- central nervous impairment in the elderly
- impairment of liver, kidney or bone marrow function
- bleeding secondary to impairment of platelet aggregation.

Use of specific cyclooxygenase-2 (COX-2) inhibitors, such as celecoxib and valdecoxib, has been associated with a lower risk of gastroduodenal bleeding when compared to traditional NSAIDs, and the COX-2 inhibitors were believed to be cost-effective in patients at high-risk for gastrointestinal complications. There is controversy surrounding this class of drug and cardiovascular events, such as worsening hypertension, stroke and myocardial infarction. Rofecoxib, recently withdrawn by the Food and Drug Administration in the USA, has been associated with an increase in cardiovascular events. More investigation is needed to determine if the increase in cardiovascular events is unique to rofecoxib or is a class effect.

Glucosamine sulfate and chondroitin sulfate are cartilage components and are available over-the-counter in various doses as nutritional supplements. Currently, their long-term benefit and mechanism of action are unclear, as the timing of improvement in pain does not correspond to the time required for their incorporation into cartilage. Over-the-counter topical capsaicin, applied four times per day, is sometimes useful in the treatment of pain. A side-effect is local burning which generally subsides with continued use.

Intraarticular corticosteroids or hyaluronic acid derivatives injections may be appropriate in some patients who have inflammatory disease, or who have contraindications to or have pain despite NSAID therapy. Hyaluronic acid is injected into the affected joint as a three-dose or five-dose weekly series. Corticosteroid intraarticular injections may be repeated two to three times per year safely over a period of up to two years. Their effect on symptoms is modest and declines with increasing OA severity. Neither modality has been shown to alter disease progression. The major drawbacks to intraarticular injections are postinjection flare manifested by pain and swelling, and risk of introducing an infection in the joint.

Surgical interventions

In some patients with OA, surgery may be a treatment option. Procedures include:

- joint arthroscopy
- debridement
- lavage
- fusion
- osteotomy.

However, the indications and effectiveness of these interventions are unclear. In those with significant disability due to OA and advanced radiographic disease, joint replacement should be considered as an intervention that commonly has a dramatic effect on quality of life.

Conclusion

In summary, OA is a disease that disproportionately affects post-menopausal women. Age is the strongest risk factor for developing OA and the effects of oestrogen on the disease are unclear. The disease is characterized by cartilage loss and, often, pain and radiographic changes. Both pharmacologic and nonpharmocologic modalities are treatment options and include weight loss, and physical and occupational therapy, over-the-counter NSAIDs, prescription drugs and surgery.

Further reading

Cicuttini FM, Spector T, Baker J. Risk factors for osteoarthritis in the tibiofemoral and patellofemoral joints of the knee. *J Rheumatol* 1997; **24**: 1164–7.

DeGroot J, Verzijl N, Bank RA *et al.* Age-related decrease in proteoglycan synthesis of human articular chondrocytes: the role of nonenzymatic glycation. *Arthritis Rheum* 1999; **42**: 1003–9.

Felson DT, McLaughlin S, Goggins J *et al.* Bone marrow edema and its relation to progression of knee osteoarthritis. *Ann Intern Med* 2003; **139**: 330–6.

Felson DT, Naimark A, Anderson J *et al.* The prevalence of knee osteoarthritis in the elderly. The Framingham Osteoarthritis Study. *Arthritis Rheum* 1987; **30**: 914–18.

Felson DT, Zhang Y, Hannan M *et al.* Risk factors for incident radiographic knee osteoarthritis in the elderly. *Arthritis Rheum* 1997; **40**: 728–33.

Fernandez-Madrid F, Karvonen RL, Teitge RA *et al.* MR features of osteoarthritis of the knee. *Magn Reson Imaging* 1994; **12**: 703–9.

Guccione AA, Felson DT, Anderson JJ. Defining arthritis and measuring functional status in elders: methodological issues in the study of disease and physical disability. *Am J Public Health* 1990; **80**: 945–9.

Ham KD, Loeser RF, Lindgren BR *et al.* Effects of long-term estrogen replacement therapy on osteoarthritis severity in cynomolgus monkeys. *Arthritis Rheum* 2002; **46**: 1956–64.

Jordan KM, Arden NK, Doherty M *et al.* EULAR recommendations 2003: An evidence based approach to the management of knee osteoarthritis: Report of a task force of the standing committee for international clinical studies including therapeutic trials (ESCISIT). *Ann Rheum Dis* 2003; **62**: 1145–55.

Kornick J, Trefelner E, McCarthy S *et al.* Meniscal abnormalities in the asymptomatic population at MR imaging. *Radiology* 1990; **177**: 463–5.

Lawrence R, Helmick C, Arnett F *et al.* Estimates of the prevalence of arthritis and selected musculoskeletal disorders in the United States. *Arthritis Rheum* 1998; **41**: 778–99.

Loeser RF, Shanker G, Carlson CS *et al.* Reduction in the chondrocyte response to insulin-like growth factor 1 in aging and osteoarthritis: studies in a non-human primate model of naturally occurring disease. *Arthritis Rheum* 2000; **43**: 2110–20.

Maetzel A, Krahn M, Naglie G. The cost effectiveness of rofecoxib and celecoxib in patients with osteoarthritis or rheumatoid arthritis. *Arthritis Rheum* 2003; **49**: 283–92.

Nevitt MC, Cummings SR, Lane NE *et al.* Association of estrogen replacement therapy with the risk of osteoarthritis of the hip in elderly white women. *Arch Intern Med* 1996; **156**: 2073–80.

Nevitt MC, Felson DT, Williams EN *et al.*The effect of estrogen plus progestin on knee symptoms and related disability in postmenopausal women: The Heart and Estrogen/Progestin Replacement Study, a randomized, double-blind, placebo-controlled trial. *Arthritis Rheum* 2001; **44**: 811–18.

Oliveria SA, Felson DT, Reed JI *et al.* Incident of symptomatic hand, hip and knee osteoarthritis among patients in a health maintenance organization. *Arthritis Rheum* 1995; **38**: 1134–41.

Pai YC, Rymer WZ, Chang RW *et al.* Effect of age and osteoarthritis on knee proprioception. *Arthritis Rheum* 1997; **40**: 2260–5.

Psaty BM, Furberg CD. COX-2 inhibitors – lessons in drug safety. *N Engl J Med* 2005; **352**: 1133–5.

Raynauld JP, Buckland-Wright C, Ward R *et al.* Safety and efficacy of long-term intraarticular steroid injections in osteoarthritis of the knee: a randomized, double-blind, placebo-controlled trial. *Arthritis Rheum* 2003; **48**: 370–7.

Ren YX, Deng YZ. An experimental study on effect of estrogen on osteoarthritis in female rats. *Chinese Journal of Reparative and Reconstructive Surgery* 2003; **17**: 212–14. (in Chinese)

Samanta A, Jones A, Regan M *et al.* Is osteoarthritis in women affected by hormonal changes or smoking? *Br J Rheumatol* 1993; **32**: 366–70.

Schiodt FV, Rochling FA, Casey DL, Lee WM. Acetaminophen toxicity in an urban county hospital. *N Engl J Med* 1997; **337**: 1112–17.

Sharma L, Dunlop DD, Cahue S *et al.* Quadriceps strength and osteoarthritis progression in malaligned and lax knees. *Ann Intern Med* 2003; **138**: 613–19.

Sharma L, Hayes KW, Felson DT *et al.* Does laxity alter the relationship between strength and physical function in knee osteoarthritis? *Arthritis Rheum* 1999; **42**: 25–32.

Sharma L, Lewis B, Torner J *et al.* The impact of gender on varus-valgus laxity in knees with and without OA. *Arthritis Rheum* 2004; **50(Suppl)**: S267.

Slemenda C, Heilman D, Brandt K *et al.* Reduced quadriceps strength relative to body weight: A risk factor for knee osteoarthritis in women? *Ann Rheum Dis* 1998; **41**: 1951–9.

Sowers M. Epidemiology of risk factors for osteoarthritis: systemic factors. *Curr Opin Rheumatol* 2001; **13**: 447–51.

Toda Y, Tsukimura N. A six-month followup of a randomized trial comparing the efficacy of a lateral-wedge insole with subtalar strapping and an in-shoe lateral-wedge insole in patients with varus deformity osteoarthritis of the knee. *Arthritis Rheum* 2004; **50**: 3129–36.

Torres L, Peterfy C, Guermazi A *et al.* Severity of pain and joint tissue lesions in knee osteoarthritis. *Arthritis Rheum* 2004; **50(Suppl)**: S344.

van Saase JL, van Romunde LK, Cats A *et al.* Epidemiology of osteoarthritis: Zoetermeer survey. Comparison of radiological osteoarthritis in a Dutch population with that in 10 other populations. *Ann Rheum Dis* 1989; **48**: 271–80.

Wluka AE, Davis SR, Bailey M *et al.* Users of oestrogen replacement therapy have more knee cartilage than non-users. *Ann Rheum Dis* 2001; **60**: 332–6.

8 Urinary incontinence: basic evaluation and treatment

Sylvia M Botros, Peter K Sand and Roger P Goldberg

Introduction

Female urinary incontinence affects millions of women throughout the world. It affects the quality of life of women of all ages and poses a large financial burden on society. The EPICONT Norwegian study found that 25% of women aged 20 to over 90 years reported involuntary loss of urine. The prevalence of incontinence rose with increasing age. The lowest prevalence was observed in the younger age groups (12% for women <30 years), the highest was observed among the eldest (40% for women >90 years). However, there was also a peak around middle-age with a prevalence of 30% among women aged 50–54 years. Similar trends have been found in other studies. Costs for treatment are high, and in the USA the direct and indirect costs have been estimated to be US $26 billion for women over the age of 65.

The most common cause of urinary leakage in women is stress urinary incontinence (SUI), which is defined as the complaint of involuntary leakage on effort or exertion. Urge urinary incontinence (UUI), the second most common cause, is any involuntary leakage of urine accompanied by or immediately preceded by a sense of urgency. Table 8.1 lists the International Continence Society (ICS) definitions of incontinence.

Pathophysiology, effects of ageing and lack of oestrogen

Continence is maintained by intrinsic and extrinsic mechanisms. The intrinsic continence mechanism is comprised of smooth and striated muscle and vascular components, all of which generate resting tone within the urethra. Intrinsic sphincteric deficiency (ISD) and low-pressure urethra (LPU) are terms used to describe decreased intrinsic urethral resistance. The lower urinary tract and the vagina share a common embryology. There are

Table 8.1
Definitions of incontinence

Urinary Incontinence: The complaint of any involuntary leakage of urine.

Stress Urinary Incontinence: Involuntary leakage triggered by physical exertion, sneezing or coughing.

Urge Urinary Incontinence: Involuntary leakage accompanied by or immediately proceeded by urgency

Mixed Urinary Incontinence: Involuntary leakage associated with urgency and also with physical exertion, sneezing or coughing.

Enuresis: Any involuntary loss of urine

Nocturnal Enuresis: Loss of urine occurring during sleep

Continuous Urinary Incontinence: Complaint of continuous leakage

Coital Incontinence: Involuntary leakage during sexual intercourse

Other causes of incontinence include urinary fistulae, diverticulae, functional incontinence or psychogenic causes.

Adapted from The standardization of terminology of lower urinary tract function: report from the standardization sub-committee of the International Continence Society. *Neuro and Urodyn* 2002; **21**: 167–8

oestrogen and progesterone receptors in the vagina, urethra, bladder and pelvic floor muscles. Thus it is not surprising that urinary problems increase after the menopause and these may occur *pari passu* with symptoms of vaginal atrophy. Increased age and decreased blood flow to the urethra, associated with oestrogen deficiency, seem to negatively impact the intrinsic continence mechanism. In contrast 'extrinsic continence mechanisms' consist of forces that help to maintain continence but are extrinsic to the urethra, such as surrounding fibrous and muscular supports. These mechanisms refer to the passive and active transmission of pressure to the urethral lumen that occurs with increases in intraabdominal pressure. Relaxation or alteration of these supports leads to hypermobility of the urethra.

The pathophysiology of detrusor overactivity (DO) leading to UUI can be divided into two major categories – neurogenic and idiopathic. Common causes of neurogenic DO include:

- multiple sclerosis
- cerebrovascular accidents
- spinal injuries
- congenital spinal cord or neural tube disturbances
- intracranial lesions
- Parkinsonism.

Ninety percent of patients with DO have idiopathic DO. Triggers for idiopathic DO include *Escherichia coli* endotoxin, bladder outlet obstruction from surgery or advanced pelvic organ prolapse. However usually the cause is unknown.

The prevalence of urinary incontinence increases with age. Ageing may adversely affect neurological control of micturition, urinary tract structure, tissue repair, elasticity of tissue and nerve degeneration. Oestrogen deficiency in postmenopausal women leads to decreased connective tissue, thinning of vaginal and urethral epithelium, and decreased urogenital vascularity.

It is postulated that hypoestrogenism affects the sensory threshold of the urinary tract in elderly patients, leading to decreased functional bladder capacities. Oestrogen appears to improve urinary urgency, frequency, nocturia and dysuria but not incontinence. Some data indicate, however, that postmenopausal oestrogen replacement may increase the risk of developing urinary incontinence.

Evaluation

History

An accurate and detailed history should be taken. Medical history alone is a poor predictor of pathophysiology. As well as obtaining a general medical history for systemic disease, medications should be recorded as they may affect urinary function (Table 8.2). Functional incontinence (due to an inability to reach the toilet in a timely fashion secondary to physical or mental handicap) and psychogenic incontinence should be ruled out by evaluating the patient's mobility and psychological motivation for continence. A self-completed bladder diary that records the frequency and volumes of micturition, number of incontinent episodes, associated symptoms and fluid intake may be useful to help refine the patient's history.

Patients with SUI typically complain of urinary leakage upon coughing, sneezing or other activities that increase abdominal pressure. Risk factors for SUI include:

- prior vaginal deliveries
- menopause
- vaginal surgery
- radiation
- pelvic injury
- obesity
- lung disease
- smoking
- strenuous exercise
- weight-bearing occupations.

Table 8.2
Drugs that may affect the lower urinary tract

Class of drugs	Side-effect	Impact on lower urinary tract function
Psychotropic agents; antidepressants and antipsychotics	Anticholinergic, sedation	Urinary retention
Sedatives/hypnotics	Sedation, muscle relaxation, confusion	Urinary retention
Caffeine, alcohol, diuretics		Urgency, frequency, polyuria
Narcotics	Sedation, delirium	Urinary retention, fecal impaction
ACE inhibitors	Cough	Aggravate pre-existing stress incontinence
Calcium-channel blockers		Urinary retention, overflow incontinence
Anticholinergic	Dry mouth, constipation, sleepiness or drowsiness	Urinary retention, overflow incontinence
Alpha-adrenergic agonists	Increased urethral tone	Urinary retention
Alpha-adrenergic blockers	Decreased urethral tone	Stress urinary incontinence
Beta-adrenergic agonists	Inhibited detrusor function	Urinary retention

ACE, angiotensin-converting enzyme

Patients with UUI complain of a loss of urine with a strong urge before reaching the toilet. UUI episodes may be provoked by environmental or psychological triggers, such as handwashing, the sound of running water or reaching home (known as 'latchkey urge'). UUI may be associated with nocturia, frequency and urgency.

Once the history is elicited, it is important to corroborate symptoms with signs, information derived from the frequency/volume chart and urodynamic diagnoses. Among postmenopausal women, deficiencies in antidiuretic hormone levels or activity may lead to excessive night time urine output (nocturnal or 'reverse' diuresis). Simple comparison of daytime and night time voided volumes may highlight this problem, defined as more than one-third of the 24-hour output occurring during the night. The use of synthetic desmopressin (DDAVP) may be considered in these cases.

Physical examination

A thorough physical examination should be performed, paying particular attention to conditions that may impact on lower urinary tract function, eg volume overload, venous insufficiency or congestive heart failure. Ambulatory capacity and mental status are assessed to evaluate a patient's functional capability. Incontinence is transient in up to one-third of community-dwelling elderly women and up to one-half of acutely hospitalized patients. The mnemonic DIAPPERS has been developed to aid recognition of reversible causes of incontinence (see Table 8.3). If a neurological abnormality is suspected urgent referral to a neurologist is imperative.

Table 8.3
Reversible causes of incontinence

DIAPPERS
Delirium or confusion
Infection, urinary symptoms
Atrophic genital tract changes (vaginitis or urethritis)
Pharmaceutical agents (see Table 8.2)
Psychological factors
Excess urine production (excess fluid intake, volume overload, hyperglycaemia or hypercalcaemia)
Restricted mobility (chronic illness, injury or restraint)
Stool impaction

Adapted from Resnick NM: Urinary incontinence in the elderly. *Med Grand Rounds* 1984; 3: 281–90

Pelvic examination

Symptoms of urogenital atrophy are commonly present with vaginal atrophy and this should be assessed. Patients with SUI without hypermobility should be further evaluated for intrinsic urethral sphincter dysfunction. A basic evaluation to screen for pelvic organ prolapse can be performed using a Sims or a Graves speculum. Thus larger cystocele or rectocele defects can be visually appreciated and, if present, referral to a gynaecologist for further evaluation is warranted. Genital tract inflammation or infection, such as monilia, trichomonas, herpes or human papilloma virus, may increase afferent sensation and lead to irritative voiding symptoms.

Urinalysis is necessary to rule out infection and haematuria. Patients with urinary tract infections should be treated prior to further work-up of incontinence. Sterile microscopic haematuria may indicate bladder or upper urinary tract disorders. Patients with sterile haematuria on repeated midstream specimens should be referred to a urologist or urogynaecologist for evaluation of the bladder using cystometry and upper tract evaluation.

Assessment of the post-void residual should be performed in all patients with incontinence to rule out urinary retention and overflow. This can be undertaken with ultrasound or catheterization. Significant urinary retention is rare in women in the absence of advanced prolapse, neurological disorders or prior urogenital tract surgery.

Urodynamic investigations usually include filling and voiding cystometry. In women with suspected UUI, changes in bladder pressure in response to bladder filling can be measured and thus help determine who has involuntary detrusor contractions. It also allows for the evaluation of bladder sensation, compliance, capacity and control during the storage phase.

If initial evaluation fails to fully define the aetiology of an incontinent woman's problem, more sophisticated urodynamic testing is indicated.

Treatment

Treatments for SUI include:

- pelvic floor exercises
- biofeedback
- pelvic floor electrical stimulation
- vaginal continence devices
- urethral obstructive devices
- urethral bulking agents
- medications
- surgery.

Treatment options for UUI include:

- behavioural and dietary modifications
- pharmacological interventions – medications
- pelvic floor electrical stimulation
- electromagnetic innervation
- sacral neuromodulation – Botox injections
- bladder augmentation
- diversion operations.

Stress urinary incontinence

Pelvic floor exercises

Pelvic floor exercises improve pelvic floor function by enhancing urethral resistance as a result of increasing strength and endurance of the periurethral and paravaginal muscles. These exercises lead to improvement of symptoms in 56–95% of patients. Patients who are selected for treatment with pelvic floor exercises should be self-motivated and demonstrate an ability to isolate the correct muscles on pelvic examination. If patients are unable to isolate the correct muscles on their own, then pelvic floor exercises with 'biofeedback' are indicated. 'Biofeedback' with auditory and visual information regarding contraction of the pelvic floor muscles improves patient awareness and correct isolation of pelvic floor muscles. Some studies indicate improvement as high as 87% with biofeedback.

Some patients are unable to isolate their pelvic floor muscles even with 'biofeedback'. Pelvic floor electrical stimulation is an alternative for these patients. These modalities isolate and contract the pelvic floor muscles for the patient and improve overall muscle tone.

Pessaries

Incontinence ring pessaries are another treatment option. One study determined that 24% of women with SUI were subjectively cured using these devices.

Pharmacological interventions

Medications for the treatment of SUI include alpha-adrenergic agonists, which act on smooth muscle to increase resting urethral pressure. Increased risks of stroke and hypertension have been reported in some patients using these medications. Tricyclic antidepressants, such as imipramine and doxepin, have both anticholinergic and central alpha adrenergic effects, making them suitable for the treatment of both stress and urge urinary incontinence.

Duloxetine is a new treatment for SUI. It is a dual serotonin and norepinephrine (noradrenaline) reuptake inhibitor that increases neural input to the urethral sphincter, thereby relieving the symptoms of SUI. Duloxetine 40 mg twice daily for 12 weeks reduces the median incontinence episode frequency to a significantly greater extent than placebo in women with predominant symptoms of SUI. In most studies, Incontinence Quality of Life (I-QOL) questionnaire total scores were significantly improved compared with placebo. In a dose-ranging study in women with severe SUI who were scheduled for continence surgery, duloxetine 80–120 mg/day for eight weeks significantly reduced incontinent event frequency (IEF), increased I-QOL total scores compared with placebo, and caused 20% of recipients to reconsider their willingness to undergo surgery. Duloxetine or duloxetine plus pelvic floor muscle training (PFMT) were more effective in reducing the median IEF than PFMT alone or no treatment in women with SUI. Mean I-QOL total scores suggested that combination therapy was more effective than either therapy alone. Nausea was the most frequent adverse event and was the main cause for discontinuing duloxetine therapy.

The available evidence suggests that *oestrogen* does not appear to be an effective treatment for stress incontinence. Placebo-controlled studies suggest it may have a synergistic role in combination with the alpha-adrenergic agonist phenylpropanolamine.

Surgery

Current surgical options for SUI include the retropubic urethropexy, bladder neck slings using various materials, and midurethral 'tension-free' slings using prolene mesh. These operations have the ability to achieve cure (dry) rates for stress urinary incontinence in 75–96% of cases. The newest tension-free prolene slings can be inserted under local anaesthesia in 20 minutes or less (patients are often admitted as a day case). Their high efficacy and low risk appear to be establishing a new 'gold standard' for the surgical management of SUI, and they have become widely implemented as a first-line surgical therapy worldwide.

The Tension-free Vaginal Tape (TVT) was the first mid-urethral tape procedure to gain widespread acceptance after prospective observational studies demonstrated high success rates. Recently a number of 'second generation' tension-free sling procedures have been introduced, with possible advantages in terms of technical ease and safety, further increasing the widespread interest in this mode of therapy for SUI. Needle suspension operations and transvaginal bladder neck plications have been largely abandoned for the surgical treatment of SUI, due to their higher failure rates and poor long-term effectiveness.

It is important for patients to recognize that UUI may persist and require medical or behavioural therapy, even if a full cure of SUI is achieved with the surgical intervention. Surgical procedures vary in their efficacy for the treatment of concurrent DO and may even cause *de novo* DO. Patients with severe SUI without urethral hypermobility are generally not favourable surgical candidates, and may respond well to treatment with periurethral bulking agents. Popular bulking agents include glutaraldehyde cross-linked collagen and macroplastique. These may be injected under local anaesthetic with quick recovery and low risk of complications, however they tend to be expensive. Subjective short-term cure rates are around 50%, but after five years only 20% of women will still be continent.

Urge urinary incontinence

Treatments for UUI are primarily non-surgical and include behavioural interventions, medications and the use of various devices.

Behavioural interventions

The simplest behavioural interventions rely on monitoring and adjusting fluid intake and diet. Review of a bladder diary provides valuable information pertaining to voiding habits and fluid intake. Limiting the intake of caffeinated and alcoholic beverages and other foods known to increase urgency can also improve symptoms.

Bladder-retraining programmes for UUI are focused on teaching the patient to resist and inhibit the sensation of urgency when it occurs, to delay micturition and to establish cortical control over micturition. 'Bladder drills' utilize pelvic floor muscle contractions to inhibit detrusor contractions through the 'vesicoinhibitory pathways' (that suppress voluntary detrusor contractions at the termination of normal micturition) in combination with mental and physical distraction techniques. Strict voiding intervals are set based on the frequency of incontinence episodes, and patients void only at controlled time intervals. The intervals are slowly increased depending on patient response. Cure rates of 18% with a 51% reduction in incontinence episodes have been reported.

Biofeedback, electrical stimulation and electromagnetic innervation

Biofeedback can resolve urodynamic DO in 44% of women, using visual or auditory signals to guide women on correct and incorrect pelvic floor muscle contractions. Pelvic floor electrical stimulation and electromagnetic innervation are also effective in the treatment of UUI and DO, with cure rates ranging from 30–50%.

Pharmacological interventions

Several medications are available for the treatment of UUI. Most are anticholinergics that act to inhibit the binding of acetylcholine to muscarinic receptors; either blocking involuntary detrusor contractions completely or decreasing their amplitude. Antimuscarinic agents, such as oxybutynin and tolterodine, are widely available for the treatment of overactive bladder and UUI. Trospium chloride and solifenacin are two agents that have recently been approved by the FDA, and a third agent darifenacin is awaiting approval. Other antimuscarinics used include hyoscamine and probantheline bromide. Tricyclic antidepressants, such as imipramine and doxepin, have anticholinergic-like effects, as well as central adrenergic effects, which increase bladder outlet resistance and are useful for mixed incontinence.

Anticholinergic side-effects, including dry mouth and constipation, may limit the compliance with some of the older preparations.

Oestrogen

Clinically oestrogen is often used to treat urge incontinence although there have been few trials. A meta-analysis of 11 randomized controlled trials in women with symptoms of overactive bladder found that oestrogen was superior to placebo when considering symptoms of urge incontinence, frequency and nocturia. Vaginal oestrogen administration may be the most beneficial route of administration.

Surgery

Surgical therapy may be an option for some women, but bladder augmentation and urinary diversion are rarely necessary. The introduction of sacral neuromodulation has provided a treatment option for patients who are refractory to medications, devices and behaviour modification. Under local anaesthesia a small quadripolar electrode lead is placed in the S3 foramina and is connected to an external pulse generator for a 7–14 day testing period. If there is >50% reduction in symptoms during this time, a programmable pulse generator is subsequently implanted in the subcutaneous tissue of the buttocks. However the procedure is extremely expensive.

Conclusion

Urinary incontinence is common among peri- and postmenopausal women, and represents an emotionally and socially debilitating condition when left untreated. Incontinence severity ranges from exercise-induced leakage that inhibits an otherwise healthy woman's ability to maintain her fitness, to nursing home admission for management of the problem and its secondary sequelae. The increasing number of drug therapies available is providing more treatment options. Experimental work with new oral medications, botulinum toxin intravesical injections and genetic engineering should offer many future alternatives for treating UUI.

Further reading

Abrams P, Cardozo L, Fall M *et al.* The standardization of terminology of lower urinary tract function: report from the standardization sub-committee of the international continence society. *Neuro and Urodyn* 2002; **21**: 167–78.

Bent AE, McLennan MT. Geriatric Urogynecology. In: Ostergard DR, Bent AE (Eds). *Urogynecology and urodynamics theory and practice.* Fourth edition. Baltimore: Lippicott, Williams & Wilkins, 1996, pp 441–62.

Burns PA, Pranikoff K, Nuchajski TH *et al.* A comparison of effectiveness of biofeedback and pelvic muscle exercise treatment of stress urinary incontinence in older community-dwelling women. *J Gerontol* 1993; **48**: 167–74.

Cardozo L, Lose G, McClish D, Versi E. A systematic review of the effects of estrogens for symptoms suggestive of overactive bladder. *Acta Obstet Gynecol Scand* 2004; **83**: 892–7.

DeLancey JOL. Structural aspects of the extrinsic continence mechanism. *Obstet Gynecol* 1988; **72**: 296–301.

Diokno AC, Brock BM, Brown MB *et al.* Prevalence of urinary incontinence and other urological symptoms in the noninstitutionalized elderly. *J Urol* 1986; **136**: 1022–5.

Fantl JA, Cardozo L, McClish DK *et al.* Estrogen therapy in the management of urinary incontinence in postmenopausal women: A meta-analysis. First report of the Hormones and Urogenital Therapy Committee. *Obstet Gynecol* 1994; **83**: 12–18.

Goldberg RP, Sand PK. Pathophysiology of the overactive bladder. *Clin Obstet Gynecol* 2002; **45**: 182–92.

Gormely A. Biofeedback and behavioral therapy for the management of female urinary incontinence. *Urologic Clinics of North America* 2002; **29(3)**: 551–7.

Grodstein F, Lifford K, Resnick NM *et al.* Postmenopausal hormone therapy and risk of developing urinary incontinence. *Obstet Gynecol* 2004; **103**: 254–60.

Hannestad YS, Rortveit G, Sandvik H, Hunskaar S; Norwegian EPINCONT study. Epidemiology of Incontinence in the County of Nord-Trondelag. A community-based epidemiological survey of female urinary incontinence: the Norwegian EPINCONT study. Epidemiology of Incontinence in the County of Nord-Trondelag. *J Clin Epidemiol* 2000; **53**: 1150–7.

Hendrix SL, Cochrane BB, Nygaard IE. Effects of estrogen with and without progestin on urinary incontinence. *JAMA* 2005; **293**: 935–48.

Huggins ME, Bhatia NN, Ostergard DR. Urinary Incontinence: newer pharmacotherapuetic trends. *Curr Opin Obstet Gynecol* 2003; **15**: 419–27.

Iselin CE, Webster GD. Office management of urologic problems: Office management of female urinary incontinence. *Urologic Clinics of North America* 1998; **25**: 625–45.

Kelleher CJ, Cardozo L, Chapple CR *et al.* Improved quality of life in patients with overactive bladder symptoms treated with solifenacin. *BJU Int* 2005; **95**: 81–5.

Kershen RT, Hsieh M. Preview of new drugs for overactive bladder and incontinence: darifenacin, solifenacin, trospium, and duloxetine. *Curr Urol Rep* 2004; **5**: 359–67.

Lin HH, Torng PL, Sheu BC *et al.* Urodynamically age-specific prevalence of urinary incontinence in women with urinary symptoms. *Neuro and Urodyn* 2003; **22**: 29–32.

Lobel RW, Sand PK. The empty supine stress test as a predictor of intrinsic urethral sphincter dysfunction. *Obstet Gynecol* 1996; **88**: 128–32.

McCormack PL, Keating GM. Duloxetine: in stress urinary incontinence. *Drugs* 2004; **64**: 2567–73.

Miller YD, Brown WJ, Russell A *et al.* Urinary incontinence across the lifespan. *Neuro Urodyn* 2003; **22**: 550–7.

Nygaard IE, Kreder KJ, Lepic MM *et al.* Efficacy of pelvic floor muscle exercises in women with stress, urge and mixed urinary incontinence. *Am J Obstet Gynecol* 1996; **174**: 120–5.

Resnick NM. Geriatric Urology: Geriatric Incontinence. *Urologic Clinics of North America* 1996; **23**: 55–74.

Robert M, Mainprize TC. Long-term assessment of the incontinence ring pessary for the treatment of stress incontinence. *Int Urogynecol J* 2002; **13**: 326–9.

Sand PK, Bowen LW, Panganiban R *et al.* The low pressure urethra as a factor in failed retropubic urethropexy. *Obstet Gynecol* 1987; **69**: 399–402.

Wagner TH, Hu TW. Economic Costs of Urinary Incontinence in 1995. *Urology* 1998; **51**: 355–61.

Ward, K, Hilton, P. Prospective multicentre randomised trial of tension-free vaginal tape and colposuspension as primary treatment for stress incontinence. *BMJ* 2002; **325**: 67.

Wyman JF, Fantl JA, McClish DK *et al.* Comparative efficacy of behavioral interventions in the management of female urinary incontinence. *Am J Obstet Gynecol* 1998; **179**: 999–1007.

9 Caring at Home

Jean Hodson

Introduction

Care at home has become increasingly important in recent years. The need for such activity has been driven not only by the current costs and pressures on hospital services but also by the needs and desires of individuals to live independently for as long as possible in their own homes. Specifically the ageing population has placed, and continues to place, an enormous strain on healthcare systems and residential homes, and home care programmes have developed in response to this demand.

In 2002 the world held 440 million people aged 65 or above, which was approximately 7% of the total population. Over the next 25 years the elderly population is projected to grow much more quickly than the total population in all parts of the world. As a result the elderly (as a percentage of the total population) are expected to increase over much of the globe, especially in the developed world and Eastern Europe. It is presently estimated that one-third of the UK population will be over 60 years of age by 2030. Under such circumstances the escalating cost of long-term care dictates careful economic evaluation. More and more evidence demonstrates that the provision of services at home provides a cost effective way of delivering care and often postpones the need for more expensive long-term residential care.

Although the aged represent the main group who benefit from care at home, many other groups can also benefit from various types and levels of care at home. Such individuals include those with chronic disability or illness, patients with enduring mental disorders, and the terminally ill in need of palliative care. In addition, there is a demand for short-term care for individuals who either live alone or with someone who is unable to assist them, and who require help during acute illness or following surgery or injury. Such care can reduce both the number of hospital admissions and readmissions as well as duration of stay.

This chapter is an overview of the wide variety of home care programmes based on medical and social services. Considerable overlap exists in the needs of the various groups using these services.

The elderly

Increasing longevity and the ability of modern medicine to cure or sustain many illnesses and conditions that would previously have been fatal has produced a large elderly population that has become dependent upon others to continue living at home. Various degrees of dependency may continue for as long as 10 or 20 years. Many of these individuals do not need or want residential or nursing home placements but are incapable of managing essential everyday activities of daily living, such as shopping, preparing meals and housework. Home care allows many of the elderly to remain at home for long periods before long-term residential care needs to be considered. Elderly individuals can be pragmatically characterized as the 'frail but well' or 'chronically unwell'. Obviously their needs differ.

Frail but well

The 'frail but well' elderly may derive support from a number of sources, but generally responsibility for home care lies with the department of social services in the UK. In other countries other agencies may be involved, such as the local hospital or even some public charities. The level of care varies enormously according to the needs of the individual, from relatively little intervention (for example a 'pop- in' service once a week) to extensive help at home provided several times a day to help with washing, dressing, preparation of meals and putting to bed. Numerous arrangements are available for the provision of meals brought to the house at low cost. These are generally referred to as 'meals on wheels' programmes and may be supervised by the Women's Voluntary Service (UK), local residential homes or other agencies. A formal care plan is agreed upon after assessment of the individual and may be adjusted as dependency increases. Private agencies provide similar services but the cost implications often restrict their use. Many of the elderly additionally derive a great deal of support from family, friends and neighbours.

Chronically unwell

Many of the 'chronically unwell' elderly need regular medical attention as well as social home care. In the past it was not unusual for general practitioners or family doctors to make routine home visits for elderly patients. However, the increasing demands of general practice, together with the changes resulting from the recent UK general practitioner (GP) contract, have emphasized more efficient surgery- or office-based care. Nonetheless home visits can still be provided where appropriate, particularly for individuals who are too ill or frail to attend the surgery. The introduction of booked telephone consultations has provided an easy and time efficient way of dealing with minor problems and maintaining contact with many housebound elderly people.

In the UK there has been increasing emphasis on the role of the district nursing team who can provide a wide array of skilled services (Table 9.1) for those needing care at home.

Table 9.1

Services provided by a district nursing team

- Regular dressings (eg for leg ulcers)
- Post-operative wound care
- Catheter care
- Insulin management for diabetics
- Phlebotomy
- Routine injections
- Stoma care
- Incontinence advice
- Pain control assessment
- Palliative care

A number of other medical services may be available to those at home including physiotherapy, chiropody and visual assessment. Unfortunately these services have limited availability and often necessitate the use of private care facilities.

Occupational therapists can organize a multitude of home appliances to help mobility and prevent falls. These include:

- walking frames
- trolleys
- grab handles
- chair raises.

Some areas are fortunate enough to have community visiting nurses for the elderly. These nurses can assess need and advise about suitable home care.

They play a very valuable role in the coordination of a multi-disciplinary approach. Sadly, financial restraints have limited these posts in the UK.

The introduction of dedicated teams of nurses, physiotherapists and home carers for management of the 'acutely ill' elderly patient has enabled many individuals to be nursed at home. This type of service, often called a 'rapid response team' or 'intermediate care team' is ideal for a usually independent elderly person living alone who develops an acute illness, such as a chest infection. Intensive care at home is instituted for a short time, usually limited to a maximum of two or three weeks. In the past this type of patient often faced hospital admission mainly for nursing care.

The future may involve the use of telemedicine. Telemedicine refers to any application of information and communication technology, which removes or mitigates the effect of distance in healthcare and is particularly applicable to sparsely populated areas, eg Scotland in the UK, Canada and Australia.

Chronic disability or illness

A multidisciplinary approach is particularly important for individuals with chronic disability. In addition to the services described above for the elderly, many have other special needs. Common conditions requiring long-term home care include:

- multiple sclerosis
- stroke
- rheumatoid arthritis
- Parkinson's disease.

Many of these patients will have restricted mobility and will be highly dependant upon nursing and home care services. They may need motorized wheelchairs, hoists, adjustable beds and chairs. Individuals with impaired vision can benefit from contact with the local association for the blind; various aids such as reading magnifiers with lights, regular loan of cassettes, large print newspapers and talking clocks can be provided at little or no cost. A selection of panic buttons or alarms is now available. These are usually worn around the neck and provide an easy method of contact in case of falls or other emergencies.

Chronic mental illness can usually be managed in the community and special home care arrangements can be put in place to review and monitor many patients. Community psychiatric nurses and social workers are assigned to these patients and provide much needed support not only to these individuals, but also to their families and carers. Domiciliary assessments by psychiatrists can be arranged where appropriate. Dementia patients require considerable support and sitters can sometimes be arranged to give family members a well-deserved break or an opportunity to leave the house.

Palliative care

Care at home is hugely important for cancer patients. This care may start following the initial diagnosis, often with nursing care after surgery or during chemotherapy. The general practitioner and practice nurses have a particularly important role to play, as patients are often distressed and frightened and have many questions concerning their future. Intervention at this stage can provide a good relationship to improve care for those who later need palliative care.

There has been enormous progress in recent years in the care of the terminally ill. It is now recognized that many patients wish to die at home and a high level of care can be provided to enable this to happen. Attention to the medical, nursing, emotional and social needs of the patient can be provided. Many district nurses have developed expertise in terminal care and some areas in the UK will also have the support of specialist nurses through the Macmillan Cancer Relief organization. Some hospices are developing 'hospice at home' as an extension of their care. The use of syringe drivers and transdermal analgesic patches has facilitated pain control at home. As palliative care patients need careful monitoring and multidisciplinary care for a successful outcome, it is particularly important that information is shared between the caregivers and the family, and that adequate information is passed to out-of-hours care teams with special arrangements for access to medical records.

Medication management

Many patients receiving care at home take multiple medicines. This can cause problems for the elderly or confused particularly when they are living alone. Poor compliance is well recognized in this group and it is not uncommon to see unused and outdated medication in patients' homes. Efforts are now being made to simplify the prescribing system and avoid waste. The key issues for successful medicines management include:

- avoidance of multiple medications where possible
- regular review and update of repeat prescriptions
- monitoring of chronic conditions with appropriate prescribing
- help for patients who have difficulty understanding or remembering medication.

Assistance may include administration of medication by a carer. Childproof safety tablet containers are very difficult for the elderly or frail to open and complicated dosing regimes can be confusing. Drugs may be prepared in daily units by the pharmacist – these are clearly labelled and easy to open. Pharmacists may operate a prescription collection service from local surgeries and a few will also deliver to patients' homes. Single prescriptions covering long time periods are now discouraged unless multi-prescriptions (to be dispensed at regular intervals) are agreed by the general practitioner and pharmacist.

Financial aspects of home care

Home care services usually incur a small charge. This varies in different areas and according to the type and amount of care. However, in addition to the care provided free or at reasonable cost many individuals needing care at home incur considerable additional charges, such as transport or extra help at home. This has been acknowledged and a number of benefits are available to help the funding of care at home. In the UK these include:

- Disability Living Allowance, which may be claimed by individuals before age 65 who have severe physical or mental illness or disability and who need help caring for themselves or have restricted mobility.
- Attendance Allowance is a tax-free social security benefit for people aged 65 or over who have an illness or disability and who have needed help with personal care for at least six months. There are two levels of payment according to the amount of help needed; the higher payment is awarded when some care is needed during day and night. For those individuals with a terminal illness, under the 'Special Rules' this allowance may be claimed quickly at the higher rate without the usual six month criterion.
- Carer's Allowance may be appropriate for carers providing 35 hours or more help each week.

Details of these benefits may be obtained from social services, local social security offices or the Department for Work and Pensions in the UK.

Preventive programmes

Apart from the recommended influenza/pneumococcal immunization for individuals over 65 and those with certain chronic conditions or disabilities, few preventive health programmes are in place for individuals requiring care at home. The use of routine calcium/vitamin D supplements or hip protectors to reduce the incidence of hip fractures has not demonstrated the same benefits in the community as previously shown in residential care homes. While there is considerable interest in falls reduction and organized physical activity for the frail or housebound elderly, the resources available to instigate this type of intervention are very limited. Similarly it is known that inadequate nutrition in the elderly may contribute to poor health. However, there are currently little objective data or funding to support routine oral supplements. Ideally all elderly or chronically sick patients should be nutritionally assessed but there is no provision for this type of intervention at present.

Carers

Family and friends provide a great deal of home care. Even when other services and agencies are involved the overall success of home care is often dependent upon the help of close relatives who deal with many of the ongoing day-to-day problems and needs. It is important that this contribution is recognized as it can be both stressful and tiring for many relatives with other family and work commitments. Opportunities for day care at residential homes or centres or short term respite admissions to allow carers to take holidays or time out should be encouraged and facilitated.

Conclusion

The expanding ageing population means that care at home is becoming increasingly important. Services and agencies and level of provision vary throughout the world. Reliance on informal care and relatives must not be ignored. Not only does it have its own stresses but it can also result in loss of employment and income for the carer, which then has long-term economic implications.

Further reading

Appelin G, Bertero C. Patients' experiences of palliative care in the home: a phenomenological study of a Swedish sample. *Canc Nurs* 2004; **27**: 65–70.

Arnaud-Battandier F, Malvy D, Jeandel C *et al.* Use of oral supplements in malnourished elderly patients living in the community: a pharmaco-economic study. *Clin Nutr* 2004; **23**: 195–204.

Birks YF, Porthouse J, Addie C *et al.* Randomised control trial of hip protectors among women living in the community. *Osteoporosis Int* 2004; **15**: 701–6.

Chapuy MC, Arlot ME, Delmans PD *et al.* Effects of calcium and cholecalciferol treatment for three years on hip fractures in elderly women. *BMJ* 1994; **308**: 1081–2.

Dansky KH, Palmer L, Shea D, Bowles KH. Cost analysis of telehomecare. *Telemed J E Health* 2001; **7**: 225–32.

Debnath D. Related Articles, Links Activity analysis of telemedicine in the UK. *Postgrad Med J* 2004; **80**: 335–8.

Department for Work and Pensions. http://www.dwp.gov.uk

International Pharmaceutical Federation. How pharmacists can encourage adherence to long-term treatments for chronic conditions. *Pharm J* 2003; **271**: 513.

Landi F, Cesari M, Onder G *et al.* Physical activity and mortality in frail, community-living elderly patients. *J Gerontol A Biol Sc Med Sci* 2004; **59**: 833–7.

Levola P, Asikainen P, Puputti M. Virtual home care of the disabled and elderly people by using user-friendly computerized virtual home care system e-Vita. *Medinfo* 2004; **2004**(CD): 1715.

Meyer G, Warnke A, Bender R, Muhlhauser I. Effect on hip fractures of increased use of hip protectors in nursing homes: cluster randomised controlled trial. *BMJ* 2003; **326**: 76–8.

Porthouse J, Cockayne S, King C *et al.* Randomised controlled trial of calcium and supplementation with cholecalciferol (vitamin D3) for prevention of fractures in primary care. *BMJ* 2005; **330**: 1003–6.

Trivedi DP, Doll R, Khaw KT. Effect of four monthly oral vitamin D3 (cholecalciferol) supplementation on fractures and mortality in men and women living in the community: randomised double blind controlled trial. *BMJ* 2003; **326**: 469.

US Census Bureau. Global Population Profile: 2002 and beyond. http://www.census.gov

10 Providing residential and nursing home care

Tom Dening and Alisoun Milne

Introduction

This chapter discusses the main issues in providing long-term care. 'Long-term care' refers to residential and nursing care homes but excludes care provided by hospitals as this tends to be short term. Although the authors focus on the UK experience, the issues raised are of wider relevance. Long-term care offers support to some of the oldest, frailest and most dependent people in society; individuals who inevitably experience multiple risks to their health and autonomy. As women make up the majority of care home residents, there are sociological and inequality issues to consider as well as purely medical ones.

The care home population

In April 2003 there were 460 000 older people living in care homes in the UK. This represents a 10% decrease from a 1993 peak of 512 000. These individuals reside in a total of 23 000 residential and nursing homes. As might be expected, the chance of being admitted to a home increases with age; for the age group 65–74 years, 1% of the population resides in care homes, compared with 4.6% between ages 75–84 and 21.4% of those aged over 85.

The world of long-term care is characterized by very old women as women are twice as likely to live in a care home than men (23% compared with 12%). Furthermore, 80% of registered beds in nursing homes for elderly mentally ill (EMI) patients are occupied by women. This reflects not only their greater longevity, but also other factors, such as poverty, poor housing and widowhood. The triad of incapacity due to dementia, living alone and limited access to community support are risk factors for entering a care home. Factors that protect against admission include:

- availability of informal support
- adequate income
- living in a housing environment which can cope with enhanced levels of disability.

Currently, there are very few ethnic minority elders in long-term care in the UK. Data from the USA indicate that a higher rate of residential care occurs in the majority white populations and this also appears to be true in Britain. This disparity may reflect the fact that the demographic profile of minority populations is younger.

Care home provision in the UK

The care home sector has undergone radical change in the last 10–20 years in most developed countries. Increasingly, provision is focused on the oldest and frailest people. Most countries have introduced systems of assessment so that places are allocated as much as possible on the basis of need. Of course this increases the average level of dependency in each home.

The funding of long-term care represents a continuing problem. In Europe there are moves to shift costs from central government budgets to local agencies and individuals and their families. Over the past 20 years, the health service and local authorities have provided less long-term care with a corresponding increase in independent providers (see Figure 10.1). The UK has also witnessed an active debate as to whether care home placements should be funded by general taxation (adopted in Scotland) or by individuals according to their ability to pay (as in England). Reflecting various changes in funding streams and regulations, the UK saw a growth in small private homes in the 1990s, but since then homes have tended to become bigger and are increasingly run by larger organizations, both voluntary and commercial. However, as the majority of places are funded by local authorities, fee increases have struggled to keep pace with the increasing costs of care, leading to an unstable homes market and the loss of many providers.

The quality of care and the vulnerability of residents to potential physical and mental abuse are areas of major concern. Most countries have developed measures to address quality. For example, in the UK, The Care Standards Act 2000 introduced a set of National Minimum Standards for Care Homes and also established a General Social Care Council to regulate the training and conduct of social care staff. Recruitment and retention of care home staff

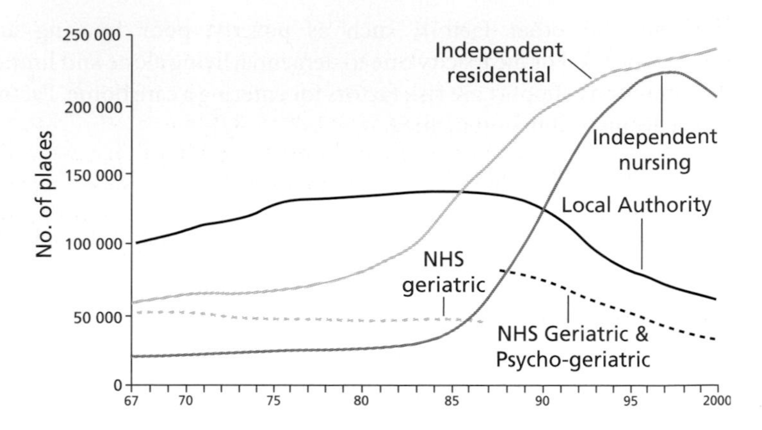

Figure 10.1 Nursing and residential care places for elderly and physically disabled by sector, UK, April 1967–2000. Reproduced with permission from Laing & Buisson, *Care of Elderly People: Market Survey* 2003)

remains a big challenge, especially in times of full employment, since other sectors (such as retail) pay higher salaries.

Health issues

Physical health

As mentioned above, care home residents are a very frail group, with a significant level of physical and mental health needs. Prevalence rates of chronic illnesses and disabilities are high and often there is evidence of unmet need or inadequate care. For example, although about 80% of residents have some degree of hearing impairment, care staff only recognize the problem in a minority of instances and provision of hearing aids is consequently low. In one study, around 9% of residents had diabetes but fewer than half of these were regularly reviewed by a GP or practice nurse. Complications of diabetes are common, and one American study found that on admission over half the diabetic residents were in pain. Care home residents are at higher risk of requiring hospital admission than older individuals living in the community, especially for injuries. The risk of hip fractures is increased four-fold and outcomes in hospital are worse, with almost three times the risk of death during admission.

Multiple physical problems and/or comorbidity with mental disorders are common. For example, a survey of 16 000 people in care homes showed that medical conditions and associated disability were responsible for admission, rather than non-specific frailty or social needs. In this sample, 27% were immobile, confused and incontinent. Although residential and nursing homes are regarded as catering for distinct client groups, with the latter caring for more physically frail residents, in practice there is considerable overlap. Both types of home contain residents with high levels of disability and need for physical care. This overlap may result from changes in residents' physical health after admission to the home, but there may also be inconsistencies in the assessments that are made prior to admission. It also calls into question the validity of the distinction between residential and nursing care.

Dementia and depression

Several studies show that over 50% of residents have dementia or significant cognitive impairment, even in homes that do not provide specialist dementia care. Many residents with dementia have behavioural disturbances, especially:

- activity disturbances (agitation)
- aggression
- psychosis
- depressed mood.

In one large study, over 90% of residents exhibited at least one behavioural disturbance. Because problems related to cognitive impairment are so prevalent, it can be argued that dementia care is the primary focus of care home provision. Unfortunately in nursing homes, staff assessments of the presence of dementia may be inaccurate, and there may be perverse incentives not to identify it, as the condition could require a more expensive placement.

Depression is also common in care homes. It is difficult to assess mood in people with severe dementia but, among non-demented residents, up to 40% may have depressive symptoms. Although most do not exhibit major depressive disorders, depressive symptoms may persist for years or until death. Lack of family support, presence of physical disability (especially pain and visual problems) and restricted personal autonomy (such as access to a toilet or to the outside) appear to be important risk factors.

Although dementia and depression are the commonest mental health problems, other disorders may be present too. Anxiety symptoms are also common, although their severity varies and they may be symptomatic of other disorders, such as depression or physical illness. Additionally, a small but significant group of residents has long-term psychiatric illness, such as schizophrenia or bipolar mood disorder.

Health services for care home residents

The provision of general or family practice support to homes is uneven and concerns are frequently raised about the quality of service provided. In 2003

Fahey *et al* found that nursing home residents fared worse than individuals living in their own homes on several explicit quality indicators. Specifically, they were:

- less likely to be prescribed beneficial drugs (eg beta-blockers after myocardial infarction)
- more likely to receive potentially harmful drugs (eg antipsychotics and laxatives)
- less likely to have their blood pressure monitored in the presence of either heart disease, hypertension or diabetes.

Unfortunately development of primary care to support care homes has been piecemeal. A minority of homes, more often nursing or larger homes, may pay general practitioners directly for their services to residents. Even in the absence of such a contract, they may encourage residents to register with certain surgeries. Other homes try to maintain continuity of primary care resulting in residents being registered with several practices, some of which may be a good distance away. Where more formal arrangements with primary care exist, regular medical sessions may be held, although the presence of such a contract is no guarantee that these sessions will occur. Limited evidence is available about the effectiveness of different models of primary care in homes, although clearly it consumes many working hours across the UK.

Access to specialist services is also uneven, both in terms of other community specialists, such as pharmacists and continence advisers, and in terms of being able to make referrals directly to hospital specialists, such as geriatricians. Support in managing mental health problems from specialist psychiatric teams is valued by most care homes although many believe that additional input should be provided. Advice regarding diagnosis and pharmacological management is generally more widely available than advice about behavioural or psychological approaches. Training for care home staff can be very valuable, but sometimes it is unclear which agency should provide the resources. Care staff turnover is often rapid, so the impact of training may be short-lived, unless managers are also involved.

Towards quality long-term care

Most care home research emphasizes its negative aspects. Despite current policy emphasis on standards, quality of care differs markedly and moving into a care home is rarely regarded as a positive choice – it is more of a residual option. However, despite a relative paucity of good research, there is sufficient evidence to indicate how care homes can promote, maintain or advance the health and quality of life of residents.

Measures that promote good care in general have been shown to be of considerable benefit. For example, health promotion, such as good diet and exercise, has the capacity not only to enhance well being, but also to reduce levels of deterioration. Evidence also suggests that quality of life for both mentally and physically frail residents can be promoted by good quality individualized care and that care home staff can play a key role in:

- enabling residents to maintain their sense of self
- communicating verbally and non verbally
- having meaningful activity and interaction.

Recent investments by some care homes in 'dementia care mapping' (DCM) – an operational model for delivering person-centred care to residents with dementia – has resulted in improvements in both the care environment and care outcomes for individuals.

Although some care homes do invest in specialist training such as DCM, the 'care role' tends to be regarded in rather narrow terms – help with activities of daily living and physical care – rather than as a therapeutic role or work involving looking at all the needs of the person. Furthermore, care workers remain poorly paid and of low status and the complexity of their role is largely unrecognized. National nursing shortages raise particular difficulties for nursing homes. Recognition of mental health needs can be improved by use of standardized assessments, for example the Camberwell Assessment of Need for the Elderly (CANE). This ensures that all the relevant domains of the individual are looked at, including mental health. Guidance for improving health care in general (Royal College of Physicians, 2000), and mental health care in particular (American Geriatrics Society, 2003), is also available.

Treatment of mental health problems

Various treatment approaches are available for behaviour problems associated with dementia – current guidance recommends that non-pharmacological measures should be used initially. Several approaches, including behavioural management, multidisciplinary interventions and aromatherapy, are modestly effective. Validation therapy and multisensory stimulation (also known as Snoezelen) may also be helpful. However, the effects of such interventions may be relatively non-specific and the impact may be short-lived. Despite concerns about possible over-prescribing, drug treatments have a role in the management of agitation and psychotic symptoms in dementia. Most commonly, low doses of antipsychotic drugs are used. Further caution is required, as there is a reported increased risk of cerebrovascular events with the newer antipsychotics.

Depression in care home residents warrants more attention. It is probably often overlooked. When it is recognized it tends to be treated with anxiolytics and hypnotics although recent work shows that antidepressants are now being prescribed more extensively. Research to evaluate the effectiveness and outcomes of antidepressant prescribing in care home settings is lacking and there is no evidence that vigorous treatment improves residents' quality of life. It probably does not increase life expectancy either and may produce side-effects that result in falls. Nonetheless, it does appear that efforts to detect and treat depression in care homes may be fruitful. Psychosocial interventions appear to have a positive, but non-specific, effect.

Conclusion

Care homes need good working relationships with primary care and with local specialist health services. They also need to work with relatives as these people may be a helpful source of information about residents as well as the providers of constructive criticism. Residential homes will have much need of community nursing input from primary care. Medication reviews, often by community pharmacists, are valuable, especially in relation to promoting more appropriate use of antipsychotic drugs. Both residential and nursing homes need to work with local specialist health services, particularly mental health services. It is not yet clear what represents the most effective system of liaison – most interventions do not require direct specialist input but mental health staff are often involved in consultation, supervision and training of staff in the recognition, treatment and prevention of psychiatric morbidity and in the promotion of health and well being.

To conclude, the present UK government has emphasized issues around citizenship and social inclusion. Older people living in care homes are particularly at risk of marginalization, but, as the authors have highlighted, there is a lot that can be done to reduce this risk.

Further reading

American Geriatrics Society/American Association for Geriatric Psychiatry. Consensus statement on improving the quality of mental health care in US nursing homes: management of depression and behavioral symptoms associated with dementia. *J Am Geriat Soc* 2003; **51**: 1287–98.

Audit Commission. *Forget Me Not: Mental Health Services for Older People.* London: Audit Commission 2000.

Audit Commission. *Forget Me Not: Developing Mental Health Services for Older People in England.* London: Audit Commission 2002.

Bowman C, Whistler J, Ellerby M. A national census of care home residents. *Age Ageing* 2004; **33**: 561–6.

Brodaty H, Draper B, Saab D *et al.* Psychosis, depression and behavioural disturbances in Sydney nursing home residents: prevalence and predictors. *Int J Geriat Psych* 2001; **16**: 504–12.

Brooker D. Maintaining quality in dementia care practice. In Adams T, Manthorpe J (Eds) *Dementia Care*. London: Arnold 2003.

Counsel & Care. *The Complete Care Home Guide*. London: Counsel & Care 2004.

Dalley G, Unsworth L, Keightly D *et al. How Do We Care? The Availability of Registered Care Homes and Children's Homes in England and their Performance against National Minimum Standards 2002-03*. London: National Care Standards Commission 2004.

Dalley G, Denniss M. *Trained to Care? The Skills and Competencies of Care Assistants in Homes for Older People*. London: Centre for Policy on Ageing 2001.

Department of Health. *Fit for the Future? National Required Standards for Residential and Nursing Homes for Older People.* London: Department of Health 1999.

Fahey T, Montgomery AA, Barnes J, Protheroe J. Quality of care for elderly residents in nursing homes and elderly people living at home: controlled observational study. *BMJ* 2003; **326**: 580–3.

H M Government. *With Respect to Old Age: The Report to the Royal Commission on Long-Term Care*. London: The Stationery Office 1999.

Laing & Buisson. *Care of Elderly People: Market Survey 2003*. London: Laing & Buisson 2003.

Melzer D, McWilliams B, Brayne C *et al.* Profile of disability in elderly people: estimates from a longtitudinal population study. *BMJ* 1999; **318**: 1108–11.

Milne A, Hatzidimitriadou E, Chryssanthopoulou C, Owen T. *Caring in Later Life: Reviewing the Role of Older Carers*. London: Help the Aged, 2001.

Milne A, Williams J. Meeting the mental health needs of older women: taking social inequality into account. *Ageing Soc* 2000; **20**: 699–723.

Netten A, Darton R, Curtis L. *Self Funded Admissions to Care Homes. Research Report 159*. London: Department of Work & Pensions, 2002.

Office for National Statistics. *UK Census 2001*. London: The Stationery Office, 2003.

Orrell M, Hancock G (Eds). *CANE: The Camberwell Assessment of Needs for the Elderly*. London: Gaskell, 2004.

Peace S, Kellaher L, Willcocks D. *Re-evaluating Residential Care.* Buckinghamshire: Open University Press, 1997.

Rothera I, Jones R, Harwood R *et al.* Health status and assessed need for a cohort of older people admitted to nursing and residential homes. *Age Ageing* 2003; **32**: 303–9.

Royal College of Physicians, Royal College of Nursing & British Geriatrics Society. *The Health Care of Older People in Care Homes.* London: Royal College of Physicians, 2000.

Seabrooke V, Milne A. *Culture and Care in Dementia: A Study of the Asian Community in North West Kent.* London: Mental Health Foundation, 2004.

Snowden M, Sato K, Roy-Byrne P. Assessment and treatment of nursing home residents with depression or behavioral symptoms associated with dementia: a review of the literature. *J Am Geriat Soc* 2003; **51**: 1305–17.

Tester S, Hubbard G, Downs M *et al.* Frailty and institutional life. In: Walker A, Hennessy HC (Eds.) *Growing Older: Quality of Life in Old Age*. Buckinghamshire: Open University Press, 2004.

Index

Page references to *figures, tables and boxes* are shown in *italics*